GUIDELINES TO
TRANSFUSION PRACTICES

GUIDELINES TO TRANSFUSION PRACTICES

First Edition
1980

Editor

Klaus Mayer, MD
Memorial Sloan-Kettering Cancer Center
New York, New York

Prepared by

The Committee on Transfusion Practices

AMERICAN ASSOCIATION OF BLOOD BANKS

1828 L Street, NW, Suite 608
Washington, DC 20036

Mention of specific commercial products or equipment in this publication does not represent an endorsement of such products by the American Association of Blood Banks, nor does it necessarily indicate a preference for those products over other similar competitive products.

Efforts are made to have publications of the AABB consistent in regard to acceptable practices. However, as new developments in the practice and technology of blood banking occur, the Committee on Standards recommends changes when indicated from available information. It is not possible to revise each publication at the time each change is adopted. Thus, it is essential that the most recent edition of the Standards for Blood Banks and Transfusion Services be used as the ultimate reference in regard to current acceptable practices.

Copyright © by American Association of Blood Banks 1980

American Association of Blood Banks
National Office, Suite 608
1828 L Street, N.W.
Washington, D.C. 20036

Edited by Klaus Mayer, MD
Editorial Assistance by Rosanne Sheehan

ISBN 0-914404-52-0
First Printing
Printed in the United States of America

Prepared by

THE COMMITTEE ON TRANSFUSION PRACTICES

of the

AMERICAN ASSOCIATION OF BLOOD BANKS

Editor: Klaus Mayer, MD

Co-Editors: Lewellys F. Barker, MD
               Anthony F. H. Britten, MD
               John T. Crosson, MD
               E. Arthur Dreskin, MD
               Dennis Goldfinger, MD
               Clareyse Nelson, MT(ASCP)SBB
               Lawrence D. Petz, MD
               Lilian M. Reich, MD
               Julian B. Schorr, MD
               David E. Smith, MD
               R. Thomas Solis, MD
               David E. Willett, JD
               Harold A. Wurzel, MD

CONTENTS

JULIAN B. SCHORR, MD, Norfolk, Virginia

DENNIS GOLDFINGER, MD, Cedars-Sinai Medical Center,
    Los Angeles, California

      LILIAN M. REICH, MD, Memorial Hospital for Cancer and
      Allied Diseases, New York, New York

      DAVID E. WILLETT, JD, Hassard, Bonnington, Rogers and
      Huber, San Francisco, California

PREFACE

BLOOD TRANSFUSION has become a necessity in the modern practice of medicine. The ready availability of blood and blood components has made open-heart surgery, radical cancer surgery, and other extended surgical technics possible. The great success in recent years of cytotoxic therapy of disseminated cancer and leukemia never would have been achieved were it not for transfusion of red cells and platelets. Dialysis and tissue transplantation would be unthinkable without transfusions. Many more burn patients would succumb to their injuries, and the survival rate of hemophiliacs would be greatly reduced. Surgery on hemophiliacs for crippling hemarthroses never would have been tried without the availability of Factor VIII for transfusion.

Because the transfusion of blood, its components, and derivatives has become essential in the management of many serious diseases, it has assumed increasing significance and is receiving much greater attention from health planners, third party providers, and the public. In fact, we now have a National Blood Policy, which defines blood as a valuable national resource. The proper use of a limited national blood supply has become a major concern to health professionals. The use of peer review processes on blood utilization has become, therefore, increasingly popular and has resulted in a universal proclivity toward blood conservation and limited medically-justified use.

In order to make full use of transfusion therapy, but to restrict its use to where medically needed, the American Association of Blood Banks appointed a Committee on Transfusion Practices. We, as a Committee, developed guidelines on how transfusion therapy can be practiced in a judicious, prudent, and professional manner. The guidelines were developed not only from theoretical knowledge, but also from a broad base of experience. Members of the Committee come from all parts of the United States and are representatives of different medical specialties and professional environments. While our views are discordant regarding detailed aspects of transfusion practices, we are of one mind in our belief that too much blood is being transfused today. As a committee of a national organization, we can develop only broad general guidelines with reasonably universal applications. Implementation must be carried out on a local basis, according to local needs, professional resources, professional preference, and custom.

We have pinpointed the locus of responsibility on the hospital transfusion service medical director. Working with the professional staff, his knowledge and experience are keys to good transfusion practices. To be most effective, he must be heard and heeded. To be successful, he must have authority and must have the support of his colleagues. A hospital transfusion committee may serve as a time-tested vehicle for communication with colleagues in related specialties. It is also a mechanism for developing support through involvement by other physicians. For this reason, considerable space has been devoted to the function of the hospital transfusion service, its medical director, and the transfusion committee. Transfusion committees can be helpful in teaching good practice and can contribute to surveillance and true nongovernment-imposed peer review to assure the best care for our patients.

AABB's Transfusion Practices Committee acknowledges that this book presents not only factual and medically-accepted information, but also personal views and opinions, some of which may be controversial. We ask only that where we make sense our views be adopted. We are open to comment, and if proved wrong, we will make corrections. We are aware, also, that there are accepted practices which are not supported by good scientific data or clinical experience. We are eager to debunk "old wives tales," and are very frustrated by the relative paucity of good, creditable, and published data on the indications for transfusion. More research and reporting of good prospective studies in this field are urgently needed. We appreciate the unresolved problems; we seek further thought and experimental work to find solutions; but, in the meantime, we advocate the most rational, experience-proven and patient-tested approach to transfusion therapy.

The Committee is grateful to the AABB Board of Directors for its encouragement and support. This work could not have been completed without the excellent staff assistance of Miss Lois James of the AABB National Office. We also greatly appreciate the efforts of our many colleagues who reviewed and critiqued this publication.

Klaus Mayer, MD
Editor
Chairman, AABB Committee on
Transfusion Practices

ORGANIZATION, FUNCTIONS, RESPONSIBILITIES AND ACCOUNTABILITY OF THE HOSPITAL TRANSFUSION SERVICE AND ITS MEDICAL DIRECTOR

Klaus Mayer, MD

Introduction

THE ULTIMATE and overriding goal of a hospital transfusion service must be to provide blood and blood products in sufficient quantities to patients in need. Since the vast majority of blood transfusions occur in hospitals, this chapter will focus almost entirely on the organization, functions, and responsibilities of a hospital transfusion service. A means to ensure accountability by the transfusion service and its medical director will also be discussed.*

The authors have chosen to use the term *transfusion service* rather than blood bank to describe any hospital-based facility concerned with the transfusion of blood. The term blood bank pertains only to the storage phase in the process of selecting and transfusing compatible blood and neglects other aspects of the management of transfusion therapy. Some hospitals combine the two terms in order to avoid confusion.

This chapter deals with definitions—often impractical or unattainable in the hospital setting—of a comprehensive and ideal hospital transfusion service, including its organization, functions and responsibilities. It should be emphasized that a hospital transfusion service that relies on a regional blood center for its blood and blood products should share its resources and expertise at the regional level. While regional center personnel often play essential roles in supplying blood, the patient's physician and the medical director of the hospital transfusion service make the ultimate decisions in assessing the patient's qualitative and quantitative blood needs.

Organization of the Hospital Transfusion Service

Every hospital transfusion service must be supervised by an individual formally designated as the medical director. This individual must be a

---

*Functions and responsibilities of the medical director are briefly outlined in AABB's *Standads for Blood Banks and Transfusion Services*, ed 9, pp 1-2.

licensed physician, preferably with board certification or with equivalent training or experience. Advanced training in immunohematology is highly desirable. If required, the individual must be licensed by the appropriate governmental agency.

Medical directors of most hospital transfusion services often have additional laboratory and clinical responsibilities, and thus are unable to devote their total professional efforts to blood transfusion problems. Therefore, transfusion service directors may choose to consult medical personnel at the regional blood center or other experienced hospital physicians when they have insufficient expertise in certain specialized areas of transfusion practice. Conversely, the hospital transfusion service medical director may serve as a consultant to the region.

Since the major purpose of the hospital transfusion service is to provide blood and blood products for the treatment of patients, and since all administrative decisions ultimately impinge on the character and supply of these products, the medical director must be responsible for the supervision, management and coordination of all transfusion service activities within the hospital. Assisting the medical director in these duties are administrative and technical personnel.

Hospital transfusion service personnel should participate in all activities in the hospital relating to the preparation and transfusion of blood products. The organization of the transfusion service must reflect this wide-ranging role. For example, it is highly desirable that the transfusion service medical director train and supervise a team in the hospital to collect blood specimens and transfuse blood and blood products. Through the work of such a skilled transfusion team, errors in patient identification can be minimized, patients can be easily surveilled, and transfusion reactions can be more readily identified.

Functions of the Hospital Transfusion Service Medical Director

Before listing all possible functions of the transfusion service medical director, two points must be emphasized. First, the medical director should be considered a consultant in transfusion therapy and in managing complications relating to transfusion. As a consultant, the medical director must actively participate in clinical decisions relating to transfusion therapy. He must develop an image of authority and should stimulate others to seek out his advice. Second, according to current concepts of transfusion therapy, blood and blood products must be requested rather than ordered from the hospital transfusion service.

The functions of the transfusion service medical director can be grouped into four categories: (1) clinical consultation; (2) administration;

(3) laboratory (technical); (4) education and training. These functions are most properly discharged by a physician. Clinical consultation must always be performed by a physician, either the transfusion service medical director or a similarly experienced physician in the hospital. While, in many cases, the directors of small hospital transfusion services rely on a regional blood supplier for extensive support, clinical consultation is best accomplished at the hospital level. Here, the transfusion service medical director has an established and continuing relationship with the physician caring for the patient, and is physically present to render advice and support. Because of greater available resources, the education and training of transfusion service personnel often can be best accomplished at the regional level.

The following is a list of the four major functions of a transfusion service medical director enumerating the tasks and activities applicable to each function. Although the list outlines possible functions of the transfusion service medical director, it is understood that many of the activities can be accomplished by personnel operating under his supervision.

(1) Clinical Consultation
- (a) All aspects of the transfusion of blood and blood products.
- (b) Both clinical and laboratory aspects of adverse reactions to blood and blood products.
- (c) Coagulation problems, including problems associated with massive transfusion, and their treatment with blood and blood components.
- (d) Special problems associated with neonatal and pediatric transfusion, including exchange transfusion.
- (e) Rh prophylaxis.
- (f) Blood volume expansion, including the use of volume expanders other than those derived from blood.
- (g) Posttransfusion hepatitis and other diseases transmitted by blood transfusion.
- (h) Clinical indications for the transfusion of leukocytes, platelets, and frozen red blood cells.
- (i) The use of plasmapheresis as a therapeutic modality.
- (j) The safety and well-being of blood, plasma, and white blood cell donors.
- (k) The diagnosis and treatment of autoimmune hemolytic anemia, drug-induced hemolytic anemia, and other immunohematologic problems which may be indicated by a positive direct antiglobulin test.

(l) Medicolegal problems arising from blood donation or transfusion of blood and blood products.

(m) The resolution of problems of identity or disputed parentage by means of blood grouping studies.

(2) Administrative

(a) Direct the management of laboratory personnel.

(b) Prepare and allocate a budget to ensure sound fiscal management.

(c) Develop and maintain adequate laboratory physical facilities.

(d) Provide the necessary and adequate laboratory equipment to accomplish established goals.

(e) Collect data and provide facilities for the storage and retrieval of records.

(f) Achieve familiarity with blood bank licensing standards.

(g) Foster innovative plans for blood donor recruitment at the hospital or, when appropriate, at the regional level.

(h) Coordinate efficient blood collection and distribution to enhance availability and optimum utilization of blood in the regional community and minimize the outdating of blood.

(3) Laboratory (Technical)

(a) Ensure the proper performance and recording of all tests carried out on blood specimens collected from donors and patients.

(b) Maintain an adequate blood and blood component inventory.

(c) Ensure proper patient identification when blood samples are collected, and when blood and blood products are transfused.

(d) Introduce and maintain an adequate quality control program to ensure accurate results.

(e) Introduce developmental programs and new products, equipment, and technics when appropriate.

(f) Develop the capability of resolving complex immunohematology problems, or seek outside consultation for them.

(4) Educational and Training

(a) Establish and maintain training programs for new employees.

(b) Ensure that the training of laboratory staff is such that they can recognize and resolve problems.

(c) Establish and maintain continuing education programs to keep employees abreast of new developments.

(d) Foster increased sophistication about the transfusion of blood products among physicians, nurses, and other allied health personnel.

(e) Establish postdoctoral programs for the training of physicians in blood banking.

(f) Introduce blood bank topics into the curricula of medical and nursing schools.

Responsibilities of the Hospital Transfusion Service Medical Director

The primary responsibility of the hospital transfusion service medical director is to provide sufficient quantities of compatible and properly tested blood and blood products, when required. The medical director is accountable to the patient-user of the blood and his physician. The blood products supplied must be the safest and most appropriate available, as governed by the clinical circumstances.

The transfusion service medical director is responsible for providing blood products for all of the patients in a hospital. He has, thus, a total overview of blood requirements, a perspective not shared by other physicians in the hospital, who are concerned primarily with the welfare of individual patients. Accordingly, the medical director must be concerned about the blood needs of each and every patient, and must not jeopardize the welfare of any patient by the disproportionate allocation of limited blood resources.

Another responsibility of the medical director is to conserve blood resources. This requires continued emphasis on blood component therapy in hospital transfusion practice so that more than one patient can derive benefit from a single donation of blood. The medical director must also guard against excessive or inappropriate transfusion or crossmatching of blood products. The hospital Transfusion Committee, in cooperation with the medical director, can provide a mechanism for monitoring the appropriateness of blood orders. Outdating of blood must be kept to a minimum.

Because the medical director acts as a consultant in the use of blood, he has an obligation to question or even deny blood products if he determines that a transfusion would inflict a significantly greater risk to the patient than withholding the product. In such situations, it is incumbent on the transfusion service medical director to confer with the patient's physician, to examine all options very carefully, and, if necessary, to suggest alternate forms of therapy. Any case in which the medical director denies the issuance of blood should be referred to the Transfusion Committee or the hospital chief of staff for adjudication. In emergency situations, if withholding blood products poses a greater risk, the medical director should provide blood products even if they are incompletely tested.

Accountability of the Hospital Transfusion Service Medical Director

Since the medical director of the transfusion service is charged with supplying blood products to hospital patients in need, he is answerable to the patient and his physician whenever blood cannot be provided or if the hospital transfusion services are inadequate. In practice, the medical director and other hospital physicians must work as a team, demanding the highest performance standards from each other. There must be constant communication between the medical director and other hospital physicians. Such an exchange of information is an informal, but effective, form of accountability.

The hospital Transfusion Committee is the most effective means to formally account for the hospital transfusion service and its medical director. This Committee, which derives its authority from the hospital Executive Committee or medical staff organization, is charged with reviewing all hospital transfusion practices, including all activities of the transfusion service.

Some hospitals have replaced the Transfusion Committee with a Medical Audit Committee, which regularly reviews various aspects of hospital care, including transfusion practices. The Medical Audit Committee is, in some respects, completely interchangeable with a Transfusion Committee. However, the members of a Transfusion Committee are often selected for their interest in blood transfusion and there may not be a similar level of interest among Medical Audit Committee members. Moreover, medical audits are often more concerned with outcome than process.

The membership of the hospital Transfusion Committee should consist of the medical director of the transfusion service, a representative of one of the surgical specialities, an anesthesiologist, an internist (preferably with a background in hematology), and other physicians, ie, a general practitioner, pediatrician, or obstetrician who is involved in blood transfusion. A nurse, a medical technologist from the transfusion service, and a hospital administrator should also be represented. It is also helpful to include a representative from the record room, particularly if record librarians are being consulted to determine a patient's transfusion history. While it is often convenient for the same group of physicians to serve on the Transfusion Committee, the Tissue Committee, and the Laboratory Committee, such an arrangement may dilute the Committee's effectiveness in dealing with blood transfusion topics. Since many decisions of the Transfusion Committee involve medical judgment, nonphysicians should not be included as voting members of the Committee.

6

Functions of the hospital Transfusion Committee include the following: (1) educating physicians, nurses, and other hospital personnel in the proper methods of selecting and transfusing blood products; (2) establishing and enforcing hospital transfusion guidelines; (3) monitoring the transfusion of all blood products in the hospital; (4) reviewing transfusion reactions in the hospital; (5) serving as a forum for the resolution of disagreements between hospital physicians and transfusion service medical directors; (6) reviewing all incidents of disease transmission by blood transfusion; and (7) serving as a locus of accountability for the transfusion service medical director.

The educational functions of the Transfusion Committee cannot be overemphasized. The Committee should serve not as a punitive body, but rather as one which highlights and disseminates new information about blood components and transfusion technics. When the educational functions are properly discharged, the Committee will have completed the majority of its work.

It is essential that the Transfusion Committee establish guidelines covering all aspects of the transfusion of blood and blood products in the hospital. Specifically, these guidelines deal with such diverse topics as clinical indications for the transfusion of blood, platelets, and albumin; maximum blood orders for various surgical procedures; and the diagnosis and treatment of a variety of transfusion reactions. Once the guidelines are established and promulgated among the medical staff and hospital personnel, the Committee must then enforce the guidelines and measure hospital transfusion practices against them.

Another function of the Transfusion Committee is to monitor the effectiveness and appropriateness of all hospital blood transfusions. When blood products are requested, the physician should supply the following information: the patient's diagnosis, the reason for the transfusion, the hemoglobin or hematocrit, coagulation data (if indicated), and whether or not the patient is actively bleeding. This information will enable the transfusion service medical director to evaluate the appropriateness and urgency of each request at the time it is made.

A practical mechanism for monitoring the transfusion of all blood products in a hospital should be established. In small hospitals, it is often feasible for physicians on the Transfusion Committee to review the charts of transfused patients. In larger facilities, however, it is more practical to require the record room to screen preliminarily the medical records of transfused patients. This involves comparing the established hospital transfusion guidelines with the indications for transfusion supplied by the physician. Computerization of hospital records may expedite such screening. Cases in which transfusion practices are not in compliance with

7

the transfusion guidelines should be forwarded to the Transfusion Committee for evaluation and action.

Relationship Between the Hospital Transfusion Service Medical Director and the Director of the Regional Blood Program

The goal of any blood service system is to provide blood products to the patients whenever needed and in the quantity that is required. The hospital transfusion service medical director and the director of the organization supplying the hospital with blood must be able to work together in an efficient, harmonious manner. The hospital transfusion service medical director should seek consultation from the medical staff of the regional blood center when he encounters problems beyond his level of expertise. Products not prepared and services not rendered at the hospital must be provided by the regional supplier. Directors at the hospital and regional blood service units must jointly encourage the widespread use of component therapy, cooperate in inventory rotation to diminish the outdating of blood, encourage blood donation, and strive to educate and upgrade the skills of all personnel dealing with blood products in their area.

It is vital that the hospital transfusion service medical director play an important role in governing the regional center that supplies the hospital with blood and blood products. This will ensure that the needs of the hospitals and the patients that they serve are heard and respected. A Transfusion Committee should be established at the regional level to create a locus of accountability for the regional center. The membership of a regional Transfusion Committee should consist of transfusion service medical directors and other physicians of hospitals within the region. A regional Transfusion Committee has the same functions and responsibilities as its counterpart in the hospital promoting good transfusion practices and monitoring blood usage in every hospital in its region.

References

1. *Standards for Blood Banks and Transfusion Services,* ed 9. Washington, DC, American Association of Blood Banks, 1978.
2. Kuhns WJ, Allen FH Jr, Kellner A: Blood banking as a professional discipline in medicine. *Transfusion* 15:152, 1975.
3. Functions and duties of the transfusion service director and hospital transfusion committee. *New York State Health Code,* 1976.
4. Dolan WD, Huggins CE, MacNamara TF, et al (eds): In another vein: Rationale and criteria for studying blood transfusions. *Quality Review Bulletin,* 3:12, 11, 1977.

5. Friedman BA, Oberman HA, Chadwick AR, et al: The maximum surgical blood order schedule and surgical blood use in the United States. *Transfusion* 16:380, 1976.

Chapter 2

DONOR-RECIPIENT IDENTIFICATION, PRETRANSFUSION TESTING AND ADMINISTRATION OF BLOOD AND COMPONENTS

Klaus Mayer, MD

Introduction

GENERAL CONSIDERATIONS regarding the administration of all blood components are discussed in this chapter. Considerations related to the administration of specific components are discussed in those chapters concerning each component.

Blood transfusion is a complex process that almost always involves multiple personnel. Giving the properly designated donor component to the correct recipient is imperative to a successful transfusion. Hemolytic transfusion reactions usually are caused by errors in the donor-recipient identification process. The probability of such errors is directly proportional to the skills and knowledge of the team involved.

Transfusion safety is best accomplished by a specially trained team responsible for obtaining pretransfusion recipient specimens and for starting all transfusions.

If the transfusion service cannot be staffed by such a team, its transfusion protocol must otherwise ensure accurate donor-recipient identification. Transfusion requests and pretransfusion blood specimens must be carefully verified via the identification bracelet of the intended recipient. A label, identifying the intended recipient by full name and hospital record number, must be attached to the blood unit prior to transfusion.

Transfusion Request

A special transfusion request form should be provided to the physician by the hospital transfusion service. This form will help to facilitate appropriate response to transfusion therapy, providing adequate information on recipient identification and specifics on the kind and amount of blood component(s) requested. Minimal identification data includes the full name and identification number of the recipient and the name of the requesting physician. Additional data, eg, age, sex, race, clinical diagnosis and history of previous pregnancy or transfusion, may also be useful. The request form usually also includes information about location, date, time and place of the intended transfusion.

Requests for emergency transfusion must also contain sufficient information to positively identify the recipient. Short cuts and compromises are not permissible. The form may also contain a release, describing the urgent need for transfusion prior to completion of compatibility testing. This release must be signed by the physician or his authorized delegate.

The transfusion service medical director should be directly consulted in an increasing number of situations. Additional information provided on the request form will help to identify when such consultation is necessary, thus assisting the transfusion service in fulfilling a patient need. This information can also be utilized for quality control of the institution's clinical transfusion practices. As with any other request for service from a physician-directed department, the value of the request form is enhanced when it is personally completed by the patient's physician.

Pretransfusion Recipient Specimen

The pretransfusion recipient specimen must be accurately identified as a specimen from the patient on whom transfusion is requested. The specimen tube must be labeled at the bedside. Records must identify the phlebotomist. The label must include data and time of phlebotomy and must contain the patient's full name and identification number (which in most hospitals is confirmed by the patient's identification bracelet). Future development of automated scanners may change this procedure and may afford greater safety and correct identification.

When the patient is transfused over a period of several days, a new specimen must be obtained at least every 48 hours. Each specimen is identified in the transfusion service by comparing the recipient's records and by serological testing. The specimens are clotted blood samples providing fresh serum for testing. In neonates, the specimen may be venous, capillary, or properly collected cord blood.

The ABO and Rh groups of the recipient's red cells should be determined next. The serum is tested for the presence or absence of expected antibodies. A number of screening methods are used, eg, antiglobulin (Coombs) reagent. Antibody screening is accomplished by determining compatibility with group O reagent red cells, containing antigens of other blood group systems that may also be of importance. An autologous control run, detecting a positive direct (Coombs) antiglobulin reaction, should be included as part of the screening process.

If the antibody screen is positive, every effort should be made to identify that antibody. Identification can be achieved via compatibility testing with a selected panel of group O reagent red cells of known antigenic makeup. The pattern of reactions produced by these cells usually permits identification of the antibody.

Special considerations involved in peri- and neonatal transfusions are discussed in Chapter 13.

The recipient specimen is further utilized, prior to transfusion, in compatibility testing (crossmatch) of any component containing a significant number of red cells, eg, whole blood, red cell components, and granulocytes prepared by present methodology.

Usually no compatibility testing is required before administration of plasma or platelet preparations, chosen because they are ABO-compatible with the recipient. Platelet transfusion, in which Rh-positive red cells are transfused into an Rh-negative patient, may sensitize the recipient to the Rh antigen and, therefore, may warrant prophylaxis with Rh immune globulin.

No recipient specimen is necessary before administration of human albumin, plasma protein fraction, or immune serum globulin, with the exception of Rh immune globulin.

Donor-Recipient Identification

When a donor unit is issued by the transfusion service, it must carry two labels. The *donor label,* affixed to the face of the unit, identifies the donor by number, and ABO and Rh groups. A *compatibility label* or tag is also attached, specifying: the donor's identification number, ABO and Rh groups; the recipient's full name, identification number, ABO, and Rh groups; and the results of compatibility testing, if required, signed by the technologist who performed the test.

A separate transfusion record form must either accompany these labels or be included as part of the compatibility label. The record form provides the same information as the labels, as well as a transfusionist's certification of accurate donor-recipient identification and evidence of any transfusion reaction.

The transfusionist must verify that the donor identification is the same on both the donor label and the compatibility label. He must also verify compatibility testing, if appropriate. Further, recipient identification must be established by comparing data on the compatibility label with the patient's wristband. If there are no discrepancies, the transfusionist can then sign a certification of donor-recipient identification and enters a date and time for starting the transfusion. His signature provides a permanent record that proper donor-recipient identification was established.

Transfusion of Blood or Components

All transfused components must be administered through a sterile pyrogen-free recipient set, which has a filter capable of retaining precipitates, coagula, and debris potentially harmful to the recipient (Chapter 3). The component must be kept at its proper storage temperature up until the time of transfusion. Routine warming of blood is not needed and is, therefore, discouraged. No medication (other than normal saline) should be added to the donor unit prior to or during transfusion. The cellular components should be gently, but thoroughly, mixed before infusion.

The rate and volume of transfusion are determined by the component(s) used and by clinical circumstances. In hemorrhagic shock, both rate and volume must be such that circulating volume is promptly restored; this often requires pressure-infusion and a large bore needle or intravenous catheter. In anemia, it is generally unnecessary and unwise to transfuse more than two to three units of red cells per day. In general, blood should not be kept on running for longer than four hours at room temperature.

The patient should be observed during transfusion and shortly thereafter for adverse effects. Chills, fever, rashes and back pain are considered transfusion reactions (Chapter 14). The patient must be observed following transfusion to determine whether the appropriate response has been achieved. Such response is, of course, dependent on body surface or weight. In a 70-kg recipient, each unit of red cells can be expected to raise the hemoglobin 1.4 gm/dl and the hematocrit 4%. Lack of response may be the sole sign of adverse effect, and require further investigation.

Chapter 3

EQUIPMENT, DEVICES, AND INSTRUMENTS ASSOCIATED WITH TRANSFUSION THERAPY

R. Thomas Solis, MD, and Harold A. Wurzel, MD

Introduction

THE NUMBER OF INSTRUMENTS, equipment, and devices used in transfusion therapy is ever-increasing. Some equipment is used during the administration of blood components, while other instruments are used in the preparation of components. This chapter explores the impact of such equipment on clinical transfusion practice.

Equipment for Component Administration

Needles and Intravenous Catheters

Needles and intravenous catheters are available in a number of gauge sizes and lengths. Needle gauge usually refers to the outside diameter, while catheter gauge pertains to the inside diameter. In routine adult transfusion, an 18-gauge bore is generally a satisfactory size. In pediatric transfusions a "thin-walled" or 22-gauge (20G bore) needle is more suitable. A larger bore may be advisable in trauma or extensive surgery since needle bore-gauge is the limiting factor in speed of replacement. In multiple trauma, surgical placement of plastic tubing (eg, sterile pediatric feeding tube 8-10 French) in a major vein both above and below the diaphragm has been recommended.[1]

Scalp vein or butterfly needles and intravenous catheter placement units are widely used in transfusion therapy because each has a "flash-back" feature obviating the need for saline to begin transfusion. "Flash-back" refers to the visible reflux of blood into the unit when successful venipuncture has been accomplished.

Butterfly needles facilitate changing the recipient infusion set without dislodging the needle. Further, butterfly needles have a plastic handle, which is convenient for the phlebotomist. The use of flexible catheters, which are less likely to infiltrate than metallic needles, warrants careful thought in the restless patient or in a patient who may be moved during the transfusion. The dangers of infection, following insertion of long-term indwelling catheters, must always be considered. It is recommended that

15

dressing be changed and antibiotic ointment be applied topically every day. Indwelling catheters should be removed as soon as possible.

Recipient Filter Set

Federal regulations state that all transfusion products must be administered through an in-line filter. A mesh filter of 170μ pore-size is standard. The overall surface area of the standard mesh filter varies in different recipient sets. The larger the surface area of the filter, the greater the volume of blood that can be administered through the filter before clogging occurs. For blood and other components, recipient sets are available with conventional-size or large-size filters. Recipient sets with filters of smaller areas are manufactured for the administration of cryoprecipitates and platelet concentrates. Needles with filters are available for the administration of commercial coagulation factor concentrates.

The cannula of the recipient filter set should be inserted in the donor unit in such a manner that the plastic container does not perforate. Recently, filter sets have been manufactured with a blunt stylet, which reduces such a risk. The filter set must be carefully inserted so that no air enters the donor unit. Air is expelled by the recipient set itself as it is filled by the blood or blood component. If these procedures are properly followed, there will be no hazard of air embolism. The filter chamber should be completely filled to take advantage of its entire surface area. The drip chamber, however, should not be completely filled in order to measure the rate of infusion in drops per minute.

The filter should only be employed for the duration of the transfusion; in serial transfusions the filter should be changed at least every eight hours. Material that is retained in the filter serves as a culture medium, leading to dangerous bacterial growth if the filter remains in use. Both Y-type and straight-line recipient filter sets are available, each with its own group of supporters. Y-type sets are convenient when starting a transfusion with 0.9% sodium chloride solution (USP) or when mixing the sodium chloride solution with red blood cells to improve their flow rate. While convenient, this practice is dangerous because solutions incompatible with blood may be added inadvertently and the tendency exists not to remove the filter at the end of the transfusion. The straight-line filter set, used with a butterfly needle, minimizes such risks and is more economical.

Smaller filter sets, used for administration of cryoprecipitates and platelets, should be flushed with 0.9% saline solution at the end of each transfusion. This will ensure complete infusion of the components, which tend to adhere to the plastic container.

16

Pressure Infusion

Pressure infusions should be reserved for situations in which large amounts of blood or blood components must be administered rapidly. Plastic bags, which are almost universally used for the administration of blood and its components, have made pressure infusion both safer and easier. Pressure infusion can be accomplished manually, simply by squeezing the donor unit. It is more convenient, however, to use a device that mechanically compresses the bag, either by spring-loaded pressure or an inflatable cuff. The applied pressure should be no greater than that necessary to obtain continuous flow through the drip changer. Excessive pressure will cause hemolysis of donor red cells. The development of an air embolism must be avoided under all circumstances.

Microaggregate Filters

In recent years, filters have been developed which remove particles small enough to pass through the standard 170μ mesh blood filter. These are described either as "depth" filters, which consist of a synthetic fiber bed with large surface area to trap particles by adherence, or "screen" filters that consist of a fine mesh of reduced pore-size. Filters are manufactured, in fact, which combine both principles. These filters are continuously being developed in an effort to achieve optimum flow characteristics and consistent well-defined effective pore-size.

Microaggregates consisting of debris, fibrin, platelets, and leukocytes, develop progressively during the storage of blood. They may range in size from 13μ to more than 100μ.[2,3] When red cells are packed by hard centrifugation immediately prior to transfusion, the microaggregates often become large enough to be removed by standard-sized filters.[4] They can also be removed from red cells by various washing methods.[3,5] No clinically significant microaggregates have been found in previously frozen deglycerolized red cells.[5]

Most of the evidence dealing with the harmful effects of transfused microaggregates has been based on animal studies. In these studies, transfusion of stored blood containing microaggregates resulted in pulmonary hypertension, abnormal pulmonary gas exchange, and ultrastructural alterations in pulmonary capillary endothelial and alveolar Type I cells.[6-11] These pulmonary lesions, as well as obstruction of pulmonary blood flow,[6,8] were subsequently prevented in the studies by the effective filtration of the stored blood. In several studies, microemboli trapped in the pulmonary microcirculation of patients following massive transfusion[12-16] were not seen in massively transfused patients when microaggregate filters were employed.[14,15]

17

Indications for the use of microaggregate filters have not been established. It appears reasonable, however, to recommend their use when critically ill patients and those patients with abnormal pulmonary function are scheduled to receive over five units of stored blood. It is especially appropriate if the cells have been stored for more than seven days. In pediatric transfusions, it is recommended that even the first unit of blood be filtered. During open-heart surgery, stored blood should be passed through a microaggregate filter before it is administered since cerebral microembolization could result from bypassing the lungs, which normally act to filter intravenously infused material. Microaggregate filters remove platelets with varying effectiveness; therefore, they should not be used during massive transfusion when platelet-rich components are being administered to recoup a deficient circulating platelet level.

Blood Warmers

Blood and plasma components are stored in a refrigerator and are, thus, below ambient temperature at the start of the transfusion. Despite this, the recipient suffers no ill effect except under unusual circumstances, usually when massive quantities of blood are transfused in a short period of time. At routine infusion rates, the transfused blood product is rapidly brought to body temperature by normal homeostatic processes. Therefore, there is no rationale to warm blood or blood components routinely before transfusion.

Dangers associated with warming red cell components, which may be damaged by excessive heat, include hemolysis or a shortened lifespan. In addition, pretransfusion warming may introduce an additional hazard: promoting bacterial growth. A clinically significant inoculum of contaminating organisms, thus, could be transfused.

In the past, blood and blood components were prewarmed by microwave units or by immersion in warm water. Neither practice is acceptable today. Whole blood or red cells with a temperature greater than 10 C cannot be returned to the transfusion service to be reissued. Such units must be returned to the blood bank and must be discarded.

The use of an in-line warming device during blood administration is acceptable under certain conditions, eg, rapid or massive transfusion or in patients with potent cold agglutinins. A patient's transfusion record should indicate that the blood was warmed. Warmed blood must not exceed 38 C.

Massive rapid transfusion of cold blood can induce hypothermia sufficient to increase the risk of ventricular arrhythmias and to impair the ability of the recipient's body to withstand blood loss. Exchange transfusion in the infant qualifies as a massive transfusion. Some anesthesiologists warm all blood transfused in pediatric surgery so that the blood warming apparatus will be in place and functioning in the event of a greater-than-anticipated loss.

Warming devices function differently. One type uses an electric element to heat water, which surrounds a coiled tube through which the blood flows. Another warming device applies dry heat to a flat disposable bag through which the blood flows. Nondisposable blood warmers are used for cardiopulmonary bypass circuits. An acceptable blood warming device should have at least one safety device that prevents further heating of the blood once the goal temperature is attained. All warming devices should be equipped with a visible thermometer and an audible alarm to indicate temperature malfunctions.

In summary, then, blood warming constitutes good clinical transfusion practice only under limited circumstances.

Instruments and Equipment for Component Preparation

Red Cell Washers

Cell washers are used to prepare washed red cells from blood or red cells stored in the liquid state and to prepare deglycerolized red cells from previously frozen red cells.

Washing liquid-stored red cells is done to remove plasma proteins, anticoagulant, white cells, and platelets. Washing previously frozen red cells serves the same purposes, and also removes the cryoprotective agent (ie, deglycerolizes the red cells).

Washing has further been claimed to remove infectious agents, but this is better accomplished with the "transmembrane" wash involved in the glycerolization-deglycerolization procedure than by a "surface" wash alone.[17,18] Currently available cell washers employ different principles, such as continuous counterflow washing, serial batch-washing, or cell agglomeration. Solutions used in the washing protocol depend, in part, on which cell washer is used, and on the concentration of glycerol used for cryoprotection of previously frozen red cells. Recent reviews cite the advantages and disadvantages of several systems.[19-21]

Instruments for Intraoperative
Salvage of Autologous Red Cells

Recovery of autologous red cells has been accomplished by aspirations directly from the operative site during surgery. (Details of these procedures are covered in Chapter 7.) The procedure is necessarily limited to surgery where there is no potential contamination with microorganisms

19

or tumor cells. The purpose is to reduce the need for homologous transfusion.

In one system, blood (including fat and other particulate matter) that is aspirated from the operative site is passed through a filter and is returned to the patient intravenously. Since clotting factors of the shed blood have been activated, problems may ensue, eg, intravascular coagulation or consumptive coagulopathy. Heparinization of the patient may be required.

In another approach, red cells retrieved either from the operative site or from a pump-oxygenator are concentrated and washed prior to reinfusion. A recent review on the subject of intraoperative autologous transfusion discusses currently available instruments.[22]

Centrifugal Cell Separators and Blood Processors

Centrifugal cell separators and blood processors are employed both therapeutically and in harvesting specific blood components. Donor cytapheresis (plateletpheresis, and leukapheresis) permits platelet and/or granulocyte concentrates to be prepared for transfusion while patient cytapheresis permits the therapeutic removal of platelets and/or leukocytes, as indicated. The instruments are also used for therapeutic plasma exchange.

Currently, two centrifugal instruments are available. Both separate components via centrifugation in a uniquely designed bowl. According to slight differences in their specific gravities, the individual components become layered within the bowl.

In the continuous flow cell separator,[23] blood enters the bowl through an inlet port in a central seal. While the bowl spins, each component follows a separate flowpath towards individual outlet ports in the seal. Each separated component is continuously removed from the bowl via its outlet port. The components can then be kept or returned to the donor, as desired. An effective component separation is accomplished by varying the speed of the bowl and the blood pump. The blood volume, ex vivo, is fixed and is relatively small.

In the intermittant flow blood processor,[24] blood also enters the bowl through an inlet port in the central seal. Layering of plasma, buffy coat elements, and red cells occurs as the bowl spins. Centrifugation is stopped when the visibly separated components reach the outlet port. Pump direction is then reversed and the red cells are pumped from the bowl into a reinfusion bag, from which they are returned to the donor. Cell-poor plasma can similarly be returned. The next filling cycle is started once the bowl has been emptied.

The pump speed, which governs flow rate from donor to bowl, is slowed to 20 ml/min or less when platelet and white blood cell fractions are collected. The blood volume, ex vivo, is inversely proportional to donor hematocrit and, also, depends on whether a 225 ml or 375 ml centrifuge bowl is used.

In either instrument, the separation of granulocytes requires the addition of a red cell sedimenting agent, eg, 6% hydroxyethyl starch, to the blood that is returned to the donor.

Filtration Leukapheresis

Nylon wool filters, initially marketed to remove granulocytes from donor blood, are now used primarily to obtain granulocytes for transfusion. Leukocytes, principally granulocytes, in heparinized blood adhere to the nylon fibers and can subsequently be eluted by perfusing the filters with diluted ACD plasma and continuously tapping the filters.

Instruments are available,[25, 26] which continuously pump donor blood through a layer of two to four nylon filters and then return the filtered blood to the donor. Continuous filtration is accomplished at pump speeds of 40 to 80 ml/min. Volume, ex vivo, is fixed. Since systemic heparinization of the donor is required, bleeding is a potential hazard.

Blood Cell Irradiators

Patients who are severely immunosuppressed due to transplantation or cancer chemotherapy are best transfused with cells incapable of implantation, regeneration, and growth. To prevent transplantation of transfused cells in an immunosuppressed recipient, irradiation of transfused blood products with 1,500 to 3,000 rads is recommended. A shielded Cesium cell is available, which is capable of irradiating blood components in just a few minutes. The machinery is simple and consists mainly of lead shielding and a device that rotates the unit of blood on its own axis. The bag is exposed to the radioactive source via mechanical transport behind the shield. It is then returned automatically in front of the shield. Electric timers automate the entire process. The operator must insure accurate calibration and must set the timer for the desired radiation dosage. Standards have not been developed to change the storage time of irradiated blood. A label must be placed on the bag, specifying the number of rads to which the blood was subjected.

References

1. Gill W: Volume resuscitation in critical major trauma, in *Transfusion Therapy*. Washington, DC, American Association of Blood Banks, 1974, p 77.

2. Swank RL: Alteration of blood on storage: Measurement of adhesiveness of "aging" platelets and leukocytes and their removal by filtration. *N Engl J Med* 265:723, 1961.

3. Solis RT, Goldfinger D, Gibbs MD, et al: Physical characteristics of microaggregates in stored blood. *Transfusion* 14:539, 1974.

4. Solis RT, Gibbs MD: Filtration of the microaggregates in frozen and saline washed red blood cells. *Transfusion* 14:151, 1974.

5. Goldfinger D, Solis RT, Meryman HT: Microaggregates in frozen and saline washed red blood cells. *Transfusion* 14:151, 1974.

6. Ashmore PG, Swank RL, Gallery R, et al: Effect of dacron wool filtration on the microembolic phenomenon in extra-corporeal circulation. *J Thorac Cardiovasc Surg* 63:240, 1972.

7. Hessin W, Swank RL: Screen filtration pressure and pulmonary hypertension. *Am J Physiol* 209:715, 1965.

8. McNamara JJ, Burran EL, Laeson E: Effect of debris on pulmonary microvasculature. *Am Thorac Surg* 14:133, 1972.

9. Swank RL, Porter GA: Microvascular occlusion by platelet emboli after transfusion and shock. *Microvasc Res* 1:15, 1968.

10. Bennett SR, Geekgied B, Hoye R, et al: Pulmonary injury resulting from perfusion with stored bank blood. *J Surg Res* 13:295, 1972.

11. Connell RS, Swank RL: Pulmonary fine structure after hemorrhagic shock and transfusion of aging blood, in Ditzek J, Lewis DH (eds): *Microcirculatory Approaches to Current Therapeutic Microangiopathy Basal.* S Karger ,1971, pp 40-58.

12. Jenevein EP Jr, Weiss DL: Platelet microemboli associated massive blood transfusion. *Am J Pathol* 45:313, 1964.

13. Moseley RV, Doty DB: Death associated with multiple pulmonary emboli soon after battle injury. *Am Surg* 171:336, 1970.

14. Connell RS, Page VS, Bartley TD, et al: The effect of dacron wool filtration during cardiopulmonary bypass. *Am Thorac Surg* 15:217, 1973.

15. Ruel GJ Jr, Greenburg SD, Lefraka EA, et al: Prevention of post-traumatic pulmonary insufficiency: Fine screen filtration of blood. *Arch Surg* 106:386, 1973.

16. Russell WJ: A review of blood warmers for massive transfusion, *Anaesth: Intens Care* 2:109, 1974.

17. Tullis JL, Hinman J, Sproul MT, et al: Incidence of post-transfusion hepatitis in previously frozen blood. *JAMA* 214:719, 1970.

18. Coutreras TJ, Valeri CR: Removal of HBsAg from blood in vitro. I. Effects of washing alone, glycerol addition and removal, and glycerolization, freezing, and washing. *Transfusion* 16:594, 1976.

19. Runck AH, Valeri CR: Continuous flow centrifugation washing of red cells. *Transfusion* 12:237, 1972.

20. Meryman HT, Hornblower M: Red cell recovery and leukocyte depletion following washing of frozen-thawed red cells. *Transfusion* 13:388, 1973.

21. Contreras TJ, Valeri CR: A comparison of methods to wash liquid-stored red blood cells and red cells frozen with high or low concentration of glycerol. *Transfusion* 16:539, 1976.

22. Gilcher RO: Autologous transfusion blood salvage, in Sawson RB (ed): *Autologous Transfusion*. Washington, DC, American Association of Blood Banks, 1976, p 95.

23. Kruger VR, McCredie KB, Freireich EJ: Continuous flow centrifugation in a modified centrifuge bowl, in Goldman JM, Lowenthal RM (eds): *Leukocytes: Separation, Collection, and Transfusion*. Academic Press, 1975, p 14.

24. Lathan A Jr., Kingsley GF: Cell separator design considerations, in Goldman JM, Lowenthal RM (eds): *Leukocytes: Separation, Collection, and Transfusion*. Academic Press, 1975, p 203.

25. Djerassi I, Kim JS, Suvansri U, et al: Filtration leukopheresis: Principles and techniques for harvesting and transfusion of filtered granulocytes and monocytes, in Goldman JM, Lowenthal RM (eds): *Leukocytes: Separation, Collection, and Transfusion*. Academic Press, 1975, p 123.

26. Buchholz DH, Schiffer CA, Wiernic PH, et al: Granulocyte transfusion: A low cost method for filtration leucapheresis, in Goldman JM, Lowenthal RM (eds): *Leukocytes: Separation, Collection, and Transfusion*. Academic Press, 1975, p 137.

Chapter 4

WHOLE BLOOD AND RED BLOOD CELLS

Ernest R. Simon, MD

Whole Blood

Product Description

A UNIT OF WHOLE BLOOD consists of 450 ml ($\pm$ 10%) whole blood preserved and stabilized against clotting with anticoagulant citrate phosphate dextrose adenine (CPDA-1), anticoagulant citrate phosphate dextrose (CPD), anticoagulant citrate dextrose (ACD) or anticoagulant heparin solution. Whole blood may be modified by the removal of platelets, cryoprecipitated antihemophilic factor and/or leukocytes. Smaller volumes can be prepared for pediatric patients.

The expiration date for the administration of the whole blood is determined as the last day the unit's red blood cells still maintain 70% or more viability 24 hours posttransfusion. This expiration date is 35 days after the date of collection into CPDA-1, 21 days after collection into CPD or ACD, and 48 hours after collection into heparin. Because of the potential of bacterial contamination, the expiration time is reduced to 24 hours if the hermetic seal of the blood container is broken. Whole blood is stored continuously between 1 C and 6 C until it is transfused. No medications or solutions should be added to whole blood.[1-3,4(pp 3-6)]

Indications for Use

Whole blood, as well as other blood components and derivatives, should be administered only after weighing the potential benefits against possible adverse effects (see Chapter 14, *Hazards and Reactions*). Whole blood is indicated in those few situations concurrently requiring both red blood cells and plasma. Red blood cells provide oxygen-carrying capacity; plasma supplies volume, oncotic activity and most clotting factors.

The primary indication for whole blood is acute blood loss. Other indications include exchange transfusion and extracorporeal circulation when electrolyte priming fluid alone cannot be used. Whole blood intended to replace labile coagulation components (Factors V, VIII, and platelets) should be less than 24 hours old. However such fresh blood is rarely available because component processing and testing is time consuming. Ordinarily, when such component replacement is required, specific concentrates should be used.

The indications for whole blood that has been modified by the removal of platelets, cryoprecipitated antihemophilic factor, and/or leukocytes, are the same as the indications for whole blood that has been stored 24 to 48 hours, or longer. The component separation process not only maintains the effectiveness of the product, but salvages platelets and Factor VIII, components that would have been lost during storage of unfractionated whole blood.

Heparinized whole blood is indicated when both red blood cells and plasma must be provided and citrate administration is undesirable. Such clinical situations are not clearly defined but often are seen in exchange transfusion, in patients with severe liver disease who require large amounts of blood and who may be unable to metabolize citrate rapidly, and sometimes in cardiopulmonary surgery with extracorporeal circulation. The use of heparinized blood in exchange transfusion for hemolytic disease of the newborn may be counterproductive in the prevention of kernicterus (see Chapter 13 for details).

Red Blood Cells [1-3,4 (pp 3-6)]

Product Description

Red blood cells are prepared in a closed system by aseptic removal of most of the plasma from centrifuged or sedimented whole blood. A unit of red blood cells shares an identical expiration date with the whole blood unit from which it was prepared, provided that the preparation technic ensures a final hematocrit that does not exceed 80%.[1,5] If the hermetic seal is broken during preparation, the red blood cells must be used within 24 hours. Fifty to 100 ml of sterile isotonic sodium chloride solution, USP, may be added just prior to administration to restore flow rate; no other solutions or medications should be added to the unit.

Indications for Use

Red blood cells are given to increase the oxygen-carrying capacity of a patient's blood when the deficiency is severe enough to cause signs or symptoms of oxygen deprivation or when it appears likely that such signs and symptoms will develop if a transfusion is not given. In most transfusion settings, the product of choice is red blood cells, rather than whole blood, used either alone or in combination with appropriate electrolyte solutions, clotting factor concentrates, or platelets, as indicated. The use of whole blood, when only red blood cells are required, may not only be dangerous to patients, eg, patients with actual or incipient congestive heart failure, but also represents an unjustifiable waste of blood components, needed by other patients. Conversely, it is inappropriate, wasteful and more expensive to infuse red blood cells with normal serum albumin or plasma protein fraction; when both oxygen-carrying capacity and oncotic activity are needed at the same time, whole blood is the product of choice.[6]

Red blood cells must not be infused or reconstituted with lactated Ringer's solution, 5% aqueous dextrose or 5% dextrose in 0.225% saline, as clumping, hemolysis or clotting may occur.[7]

Leukocyte-Poor Red Blood Cells[1-3]

Product Description

Leukocyte-poor red blood cells is the component that remains after most of the plasma and at least 70% of the leukocytes have been removed from whole blood. This component should retain at least 70% of the original quantity of red cells. While several preparation technics have been used, none is wholly satisfactory since leukocyte removal is incomplete and some red cell loss is inevitable. Current methods include: upright or inverted centrifugation; batch washing; filtration; the addition of sedimenting agents; automated cell processors; and the use of previously frozen, deglycerolized red blood cells.

In a recent study, the most effective manual procedure in removing leukocytes was a single upright centrifugation of 6- to 10-day old saline-diluted red blood cells.[8] Upright centrifugation of 6- to 10-day old whole blood was almost as effective in removing leukocytes, and retains the shelf-life of the whole blood unit because the closed system is maintained. Automated cell processors were no more effective than several of the better manual methods. Freezing and deglycerolizing improved leukocyte removal tenfold compared with non-freezing methods. While fewer red blood cells are lost, the costs incurred are greater using freezing and deglycerolization technics.

Indications for Use

Leukocyte-poor red blood cells are indicated primarily in patients having repeated febrile transfusion reactions due to demonstrated or suspected antileukocyte antibodies. Such reactions are characterized by an initial flush, followed by fever and a shaking chill, occurring during or shortly after the administration of blood. The febrile response may persist for four to eight hours. Occasionally the manifestations are more severe and include nausea, vomiting, chest and back pain, and rarely normovolemic pulmonary edema.[9,10] Although such reactions are usually not serious, they may be confused with hemolytic transfusion reactions. Nonhemolytic febrile reactions are relatively frequent. Several transfusions are usually required to induce sensitization to leukocyte antigens in men, nonparous women, and children. In gravid or parous women, reactions may occur with the first or second transfusion.[11]

Since some febrile reactions cannot be attributed to sensitivity to leukocytes, patients should not be switched to leukocyte-poor red blood cells after only a single reaction. A reasonable practice is to use leukocyte-poor red blood cells in multiparous women or multitransfused patients who repeatedly have febrile reactions to blood.[12] The severity of the reaction usually depends on the number of granulocytes transfused; most reactions are minimized when 70% to 80% of the original number of granulocytes are removed.[13] Accordingly, the freezing and deglycerolizing procedure should be reserved for the uncommon situation in which manual preparation methods do not prevent reactions. Rarely, leukocyte antibodies present in donor blood cause chills, fever, nonproductive cough, dyspnea and normovolemic pulmonary edema.[10,14] When such a donor is identified, whole blood or plasma from that donor should not be transfused.

Removal of leukocytes and/or pretransfusion irradiation of the unit of blood or component may be considered to reduce the risk of transfusion-induced graft-versus-host disease in fetuses, some newborns, or in severely immunocompromised and myelosuppressed recipients. However, additional date are needed.[15]

Leukocyte-poor red blood cells have been considered the product of choice when transfusing patients with paroxysmal nocturnal hemoglobinuria (PNH) to prevent possible hemolysis of the patient's own red cells. Recent data indicate that this is unnecessary.[16] The authors recommend that PNH patients be transfused with group specific red blood cells or whole blood using the same precautions as with any other frequently transfused patient.

Deglycerolized Red Blood Cells [1,3]

Product Description

Deglycerolized red blood cells, prepared from frozen red blood cells, is the component remaining after most of the viable cellular elements other than red blood cells (and some lymphocytes[17]), and virtually all of the plasma constituents of the original blood unit have been removed.

Glycerol, the cryoprotective agent which is used when the red blood cells are frozen, is usually added within six days of collection of the source blood. It must be removed by washing prior to transfusion, partly to avert toxicity but primarily to prevent osmotic hemolysis, in vivo. Currently, two preparation methods are used: a high glycerol (40%

w/v) slow freeze-and-thaw method with storage at -80 C; and a low glycerol (18% w/v) rapid freeze-and-thaw method with storage in liquid nitrogen at -150 C.[18-20]

The number of red blood cells recovered from a frozen unit is 80% to 90% of the original red cell mass. The survival and function of the erythrocytes, circulating 24 hours after transfusion, are equivalent to the survival and function of liquid-stored red blood cells of a comparable age (based on the number of days after collection the unit was frozen).[21]

Currently, deglycerolized red blood cells must be transfused within 24 hours after thawing; accordingly, isotonic saline is an adequate suspending solution. As data accumulate indicating the safety and efficacy of storing thawed red blood cells more than 24 hours, solutions that maintain red cell viability for longer periods of time will be required.

Indications for Use

Indications for using deglycerolized red blood cells are the same as for leukocyte-poor red blood cells prepared by other methods. Because this product retains fewer white cells and platelets, and less plasma than other red blood cell products, there are additional indications. These include prevention of rare anaphylactoid transfusion reactions due to sensitivity to transfused plasma constituents, particularly in IgA-deficient recipients (incidence about 1 in 800) who develop antibodies to IgA.[22,23] (While washing alone may suffice, the entire freeze-thaw-wash technic was required to prevent the reaction in one patient.[24])

Previously frozen, deglycerolized red blood cells have been used when transfusing potential organ transplant recipients and as a means to reduce the incidence of posttransfusion hepatitis.[25] Recent studies, however, question both of these indications for use. A striking correlation between increased numbers of pretransplant blood transfusions and improved cadaver kidney transplant survival has now been demonstrated; previously frozen, deglycerolized red blood cells were much *less* effective than whole blood or red blood cells in producing this effect.[26] With respect to the prevention of posttransfusion hepatitis, a recent experimental study failed to establish that the freeze-thaw-wash cycle reduces the transmissibility of hepatitis B, even when washing utilized the efficient continuous flow technic.[27] This finding is consistent with the results of another study,[28] which showed that while diluting the injected plasma to the degree achieved by freezing and deglycerolizing abolished icteric disease, dilutions even 1000 times greater did not reduce the incidence of anicteric infection. The anicteric infections were also associated with a tenfold higher incidence in the carrier state and chronic liver disease.[29] Results of a recent clinical study indicated that neither previously frozen, deglycerolized red blood cells nor washed red blood cells were effective in reducing the incidence of icteric non-A, non-B posttransfusion hepatitis.[30]

The expiration date of frozen red blood cells is three years; therefore, an inventory of rare blood types, as well as units typed for a number of erythrocyte antigens for transfusing patients with multiple red cell alloantibodies, can be accumulated. Freezing also allows long-term storage of a patient's own red cells for autotransfusion, a process that is especially valuable for multiple-alloimmunized patients.

Rejuvenated Red Blood Cells

Product Description

A rejuvenation solution may be added to stored red blood cells to restore 2, 3-diphosphoglycerate levels (DPG)—or oxygen-delivery capacity—and/or adenine mononucleotide levels—or posttransfusion survival—to those levels found in fresh red blood cells. DPG values may even be elevated above normal. Rejuvenation solutions may be added either alone or in conjunction with a cryoprotective substance (glycerol) for subsequent frozen storage. In either case, the red blood cells must be washed to remove potentially toxic components and metabolites from the solutions prior to administration. The most extensively studied solutions contain pyruvate, inosine, glucose, and phosphate, with or without adenine.[31]

Indications for Use

Rejuvenated red blood cells (deglycerolized and/or washed) have the same indications for use as red blood cells. Because such cells have the oxygen-delivery capacity of fresh red blood cells (or an increased capacity if higher than normal DPG levels are generated), they appear to be especially useful in situations where transfusion with DPG-depleted cells alone may be harmful. Investigations on this subject matter are currently underway,[31] but definitive indications have not been established. In the meantime, DPG depletion of liquid-stored red blood cells may be considered important when the usual rapid compensatory responses to impaired oxygen delivery are severely compromised by heart, vascular or lung disease. Even here, the DPG effect is almost certainly insignificant when the transfusion (into adults) is limited to only a few units. However, it may become important when massive transfusion is necessary for immediate improvement in tissue oxygen delivery in patients with cardiac or pulmonary decompensation or coronary artery disease, who sustain severe trauma or undergo complex surgery, and possible in some newborns with the respiratory disease syndrome. Such patients should not receive massive replacement with DPG-depleted blood exclusively.[32] (See Chapter 6 for a discussion on massive transfusions.)

Acute Blood Loss

Clinical Evaluation

While a quantitative determination of blood loss is difficult, an estimate of the severity of hemorrhage can be made on the basis of the pathophysiology of acute blood loss. A healthy 70-kg individual, with a blood volume of about 5000 ml, can usually lose up to 1000 ml, or 20% of his blood volume, without signs or symptoms of cardiovascular insufficiency. An increase in venous tone, produced by sympathetic nervous system activity and catecholamine release, compensates for the sudden volume deficit. Sensorium remains clear, the pulse stays normal, and the blood pressure is stable without postural hypotension. Severe trauma or pain, as well as emotions and drugs, may mitigate or abolish this compensatory vasomotor response. Accordingly, clinical signs of circulatory insufficiency must be interpreted in relation to both volume and vasomotor components. For example, the patient with hypovolemia due to gastrointestinal bleeding may have few symptoms until he sees the tarry stool; occasionally, it is the ensuing emotional reaction which produces vasodilation followed by syncope.

Once blood loss exceeds 1000 ml, signs of cardiovascular instability appear. Initially, tachycardia and tachypnea with mild exertion and postural hypotension are the only manifestations. In the supine position, the vital signs may still remain normal.[33]

When about 1500 ml or 30% of the blood volume is lost, cardiac output begins to fall. The patient demonstrates tachycardia at rest, excessive sweating, postural hypotension, a progressive lowering of the supine blood pressure, and often air hunger. If conscious, he experiences increasing anxiety and restlessness; he may complain of thirst.

By the time the blood loss approaches 2000 ml, or 40% of the blood volume, vascular shock supervenes. Acute loss of half the blood volume is usually fatal unless immediate volume replacement can be started.[34]

The hemoglobin/hematocrit cannot be used as an index of volume loss in the bleeding patient without ancillary information. Following an acute hemorrhage, the hematocrit falls only as plasma volume is replaced. The rate of volume replacement depends both on the intake of water and sodium and on the production and redistribution of new oncotic protein. The hematocrit falls rapidly at first and then more slowly; the predicted

31

reduction may not occur for up to 50 hours.[35] Accordingly, a low hematocrit between three and six hours after the onset of hemorrhage indicates severe blood loss; a near normal level after more than six hours suggests a modest bleed.

Management [3,4 (pp 7-11), 36]

The crucial issue in managing acute blood loss, whether associated with surgery, major trauma or continued hemorrhage, is maintenance of blood volume. In sharp contrast to the untreated loss of half the blood volume, acute losses of half the red cell mass are tolerated by most patients. Volume replacement, not necessarily with blood, must be initiated as soon as possible.

If the bleeding is controlled, blood losses of 500 to 1000 ml in adults usually do not require transfusion; treatment with electrolyte and/or colloid solutions suffices because physiological mechanisms for plasma volume replacement will restore most of the volume loss within 24 hours and the hematocrit will not fall more than about 10 points. Oxygen delivery will be maintained by a right shift in the hemoglobin-oxygen dissociation curve, which takes place as anemia develops and persists until the anemia is corrected. Transfusion with whole blood or red blood cell products exposes such patients to unnecessary risks without conveying discernible benefits.[37-40]

Electrolyte solutions can be used alone to replace limited blood losses, to keep the patient alive until blood is available, or in combination with blood to lessen the total amount needed. They are also safe, effective and practical for initial resuscitation.[38, 41, 42] When electrolyte is used alone to replace blood loss, three volumes of solution must be used for every volume of blood lost.

Among the advantages of using electrolyte solutions is ready availability, leading to quick and safe administration, even outside the hospital. Disadvantages include: overexpansion of extracellular fluid; loss of efficacy with respect to blood volume maintenance, if hemorrhage continues, after one to two hours of administration; lowering of plasma colloid osmotic pressure; and failure of the central venous pressure to reflect dangerous degrees of overloading. Colloid solutions or whole blood may be preferable for the elderly or for patients with compromised cardiovascular reserves since they are tolerated better than large volumes of electrolyte solutions.

Colloids, either artificial or natural, preserve plasma osmotic activity. Dextran and hydroxyethyl starch, the artificial colloids now available in the United States, may produce abnormal bleeding.[43] While the natural colloids, human serum albumin and plasma protein fraction, do not interfere with hemostasis, have few adverse effects, and do not transmit hepatitis, they are expensive.

No matter what product is used initially, partial replacement with blood products is initiated when more than 20% of the blood volume is lost. As blood volume loss approaches 50%, replacement with whole blood will be necessary. The more rapid the bleed and the more significant the associated conditions, the earlier blood products must be used. Non-blood replacement should be continued only if the anticipated loss is limited, the patient is doing well and no associated conditions coexist that make acute anemia less tolerable.

In cases of extensive bleeding, the source must be identified and controlled as soon as possible. Some patients will need surgery before restoration of blood volume is complete as the maximal rate of fluid and blood administration may not equal the rate of loss.

Monitoring the central venous pressure helps to detect fluid overload when blood or other fluids with plasma specific colloid activity are being administered; it may not reflect overloading with electrolyte solutions. The rate of change in central venous pressure is often more valuable than its absolute value. Pulmonary artery wedge pressure is more informative, but the procedure adds risks.[44] Blood pressure, pulse and respiratory rate, state of consciousness, urinary output, skin temperature and color are all valuable indicators of adequate tissue and organ perfusion, but each alone can be misleading.

To sum up, when blood or blood products are indicated in the management of acute blood loss, whole blood and red blood cells are selected in various proportions to replace continued volume loss or to restore oxygen-carrying capacity. Whole blood is the product of choice when blood loss continues. Red blood cells are preferred when bleeding has stopped or when volume replacement has been initiated with electrolyte or colloid infusions. Whole blood, modified by the removal of platelets, cryoprecipitated antihemophilic factor, and/or leukocytes is as effective for volume and red cell mass support as whole blood stored more than about 24 to 48 hours.

In the initial management of the massively bleeding patient, immediately available O Rh-negative red blood cells is the blood product of choice, in combination with the rapid infusion of electrolyte and/or colloid solutions; it may be necessary to substitute Rh-positive cells in an emergency. Remember that red blood cells and Ringer's lactate solution cannot be infused through the same intravenous line. Sterile isotonic sodium chloride solution, USP, is the only acceptable diluent for a red blood cell transfusion. (See Chapter 6 for details on the comprehensive management of the massively bleeding patient.)

Chronic Anemia

Clinical Evaluation

The proper use of blood products in the management of patients with chronic anemia requires clinical judgment to balance anticipated benefits in light of potential risks. This assessment requires both an appreciation of the pathophysiology of anemia and an evaluation of the individual patient for conditions which may modify his compensatory responses, for severity, and for etiology of the anemia.

When the hemoglobin concentration falls gradually, the plasma volume expands so that blood volume remains nearly constant; blood viscosity is also reduced. In addition, the partial pressure of oxygen in the tissues declines and red cell 2, 3-DPG levels increase. This shifts the hemoglobin-oxygen dissociation curve to the right and permits more oxygen to be extracted from capillary blood. If delivery of oxygen remains inadequate to meet tissue needs, a compensatory increase in cardiac output and stroke volume takes place. Blood flow is diverted from kidneys, skin, resting muscle and gut, to apparently more vital regions (heart and brain).[45] These adjustments are influenced by severity, chronicity, competency of the cardiovascular system, vasomotor regulatory mechanisms, and the individual's oxygen requirements (physical and metabolic activity).

As a consequence, the gradual development of mild or even moderately severe anemia does not produce tissue hypoxia or significant symptoms at rest, unless the compensatory mechanisms are compromised, or an increased oxygen demand exists. As oxygen needs are increased by physical activity or disease, moderate anemia may produce signs and symptoms which relate to compensatory cardiovascular adjustments, decreased regional blood flow and/or decreased oxygen delivery. Hyperpnea, palpitation, exertional tachycardia, systolic murmur and bounding pulse reflect the compensatory adjustments. Weakness and fatigue reflect decreased blood flow and/or oxygen delivery to the extremities; hypersensitivity to cold and pallor—to the skin; loss of appetite with indigestion—to the gut; and mental confusion, dizziness, headache, insomnia, inability to concentrate, and syncope—to the central nervous system.[45-47]

In an otherwise healthy individual with chronic anemia, exertional dyspnea will appear at a hemoglobin level around 7.5 g/dl, weakness at less than 6 g/dl, dyspnea at rest at about 3 g/dl, and heart failure around 2.5 g/dl.[46] Even though anemia reduces maximal exercise capacity,[48] many patients, including some who do physical work, tolerate chronic anemia with hematocrits approaching half normal with few signs or symptoms.

If compensatory mechanisms are impaired by diseases affecting cardio-pulmonary function or vasomotor regulation, or if oxygen demand is increased, such as by fever, signs and symptoms appear at higher hemoglobin concentrations and the risks of uncorrected anemia increase. The combined effects of anemia and local vascular disease are particularly important. Examples include coronary artery disease producing angina pectoris or heart failure, peripheral vascular disease producing inter-mittent claudication and cerebrovascular disease resulting in disorien-tation or impaired vasomotor regulation.

Patients with anemias that can be expected to respond to therapy, must be identified so that specific therapy can be initiated. Identification cate-gories include: disorders of red cell production, eg, megaloblastic and iron deficiency anemias; and disorders of loss or destruction, eg, gastrointestinal bleeding or hemolytic disease.

Transfusions will lessen the anemia and may ameliorate signs and symptoms, but the effect is temporary. If the underlying disease is not modified, the transfusions will merely suppress erythropoiesis, and anemia of comparable severity will recur within weeks, as the transfused red cells age and are removed from circulation. Chronic transfusion therapy is expensive, inconvenient, and exposes the patient to the hazards of each transfusion episode; it may also produce iron overload and elicit im-munologic reactions which make subsequent transfusion therapy dif-ficult.[49] For some patients, compatible donor blood may become nearly impossible to find, thereby increasing the risks of future transfusions.

Management

Specific therapy should be initiated for any disorder of red cell pro-duction or destruction which is likely to respond. Patients with chronic gastrointestinal blood loss that cannot be corrected should receive iron therapy to reduce or eliminate the need for transfusion. In some unusual cases, eg, in patients with hereditary telangiectasia, in some with gastro-intestinal malignancies, hiatus hernia or bleeding sites that cannot be identified, the rate of iron loss may be greater than the rate of replacement through maximally tolerated oral or intramuscular iron therapy. Here, intravenous iron-dextran may be administered.[50]

In the severely anemic patient with hypoxic symptoms, bed rest, diuretics and cardiac glycosides, when indicated, combined with oxygen administration, may suffice until the effects of specific therapy become manifest. Supplemental oxygen can provide additional dissolved O_2 in the plasma and increase oxygen delivery by 15% to 25%.[45]

When a rapid increase in oxygen-carrying capacity is required to relieve hypoxia while awaiting the effects of specific therapy, or when specific therapy is not applicable, blood products must be used. Transfusions should not be used if symptomatology is minimal or if no unusual stress, as for example emergency surgery, is anticipated. Remember, it is not necessary to correct the anemia completely; the only objective is amelioration or prevention of anticipated hypoxia.

In transfusing patients with chronic anemia, red blood cells are the product of choice. Whole blood is rarely, if ever, indicated. In the elderly, or in patients with limited cardiac reserves, the hazard of volume overload should be minimized by infusing the red blood cells no faster than 1 or 2 ml/kg/hour, administering a potent diuretic, and/or removing an equivalent volume of the patient's blood as the red blood cells are given. Such measures must not replace close clinical monitoring for evidence of congestive heart failure during, as well as following, the transfusion. Heart failure after infusion of as little as 200 ml of red cells has developed up to 12 hours later and has proven fatal.[51]

While strict criteria for transfusing patients with chronic anemia cannot be given, some guidelines should be considered. In the absence of cardiovascular disease, most patients are comfortable with hemoglobin levels of 7 g/dl and do not require transfusion. For anemias of greater severity, symptoms of hypoxia usually are present and may prove incapacitating. It is in these cases that clinical judgment is most critical. Many patients adjust adequately to their decreased exercise tolerance and can avoid the problems associated with a program of chronic transfusions. At sustained hemoglobin levels below 5 g/dl, most, but not all, patients will require transfusion.

Patients with severe congenital anemias, such as thalassemia, present a special problem. Recent studies suggest that red blood cells used to maintain the hemoglobin level at 10 g/dl permit normal growth and development.[52] Such a program will make iron overload inevitable unless it is combined with iron chelation therapy as iron stores accumulate.[53]

References

1. *Standards for Blood Banks and Transfusion Services,* ed 9. Washington, DC, American Association of Blood Banks, 1978.
2. *Circular of Information for the Use of Human Blood and Blood Components by Physicians.* Washington, DC, American Association of Blood Banks/American Red Cross, 1978.
3. The Advisory Panel for Review of Blood and Blood Derivatives, Bureau of Biologics, Food and Drug Administration, Bethesda, MD, 1975 to 1978.
4. Greenwalt TJ, Polesky HF, Chaplin H, et al (eds): *General Principles of Blood Transfusion.* Chicago, American Medical Association, 1977.

5. Beutler E, West C: The storage of hard-packed red blood cells in citrate-phosphate-dextrose (CPD) and CPD-adenine (CPDA-1). *Blood* 54:280-284, 1979.

6. Schmidt PJ: Red cells for transfusion. *N Engl J Med* 299: 1411-1412, 1978.

7. Ryden SE, Oberman HA: Compatibility of common intravenous solutions with CPD blood. *Transfusion* 15:250-255, 1975.

8. Meryman HT, Bross J, Lebowitz R: The preparation of leukocyte-poor red cells: A comparative study. *Transfusion,* 20:1980.

9. Cannon DC: Clinical aspects of the leukocyte antibody reaction. *Postgrad Med* 47:51-53, 1970.

10. Thompson JS, Severson DC, Parmely BL, et al: Pulmonary "hypersensitivity" reactions induced by transfusion of non-HL-A leukoagglutinins. *N Engl J Med* 284:1120-1125, 1971.

11. Masouredis SP: Preservation and clinical use of erythrocytes and whole blood, in Williams WJ, Beutler E, Erslev AJ, et al (eds): *Hematology,* ed 2. New York, McGraw-Hill Book Company, 1977, chap 166.

12. Kevy SV, Schmidt PJ, McGinniss MH, et al: Febrile, non-hemolytic transfusion reactions and the limited role of leukoagglutinins in their etiology. *Transfusion* 2:7-16, 1962.

13. Perkins HA, Payne R, Ferguson J, et al: Nonhemolytic febrile transfusion reactions. *Vox Sang* 11:578-600, 1966.

14. Ward HN: Pulmonary infiltrates associated with leukoagglutinin transfusion reactions. *Ann Intern Med* 73:689-694, 1970.

15. Cohen D, Weinstein H, Mihm M, et al: Nonfatal graft-versus-host disease occurring after transfusion with leukocytes and platelets obtained from normal donors. *Blood* 53:1053-1057, 1979.

16. Sherman SP, Taswell HF: The need for transfusion of saline-washed red blood cells to patients with paroxysmal noctural hemoglobinemia: A myth. *Transfusion* 17:683, 1977.

17. Telischi M, Krmpotic E, Moss G: Viable lymphocytes in frozen washed blood. *Transfusion* 15:481-484, 1975.

18. Huggins CE: Practical preservation of blood by freezing, in *Red Cell Freezing.* Washington, DC, American Association of Blood Banks, 1973, pp 31-54.

19. Rowe AW: Preservation of blood by the low glycerol-rapid freeze process, in *Red Cell Freezing.* Washington, DC, American Association of Blood Banks, 1973, pp 55-72.

20. Meryman HT: A high glycerol red cell freezing method, in *Red Cell Freezing.* Washington, DC, American Association of Blood Banks, 1973, pp 73-86.

21. Valeri CR: Viability and function of preserved red cells. *N Engl J Med* 284:81-88, 1971.

22. Vyas GN, Perkins HA, Yang YM, et al: Healthy blood donors with selective absence of immunoglobin A: Prevention of anaphylactic transfusion reactions caused by antibodies to IgA. *J Lab Clin Med* 85:838-842, 1975.

23. Pineda AA, Taswell HA: Transfusion reactions associated with anti-IgA antibodies: Report of four cases and review of the literature. *Transfusion* 15:10-15, 1975.

24. Miller WV, Holland PV, Sugarbaker E, et al: Anaphylactic reactions to IgA. *Am J Clin Pathol* 54:618-621, 1970.

25. Tullis JL, Hinman J, Sproul MT, et al: Incidence of post-transfusion hepatitis in previously frozen blood. *JAMA* 214:719-723, 1970.

26. Opelz G, Terasaki PI: Improvement of kidney-graft survival with increased numbers of blood transfusions. *N Engl J Med* 299:799-803, 1978.

27. Alter HJ, Tabor E, Meryman HT, et al: Transmission of hepatitis B virus infection by transfusion of frozen-deglycerolized red blood cells. *N Engl J Med* 298:637-642, 1978.

28. Barker LF, Murray R: Relationship of virus dose to incubation time of clinical hepatitis and time of appearance of hepatitis-associated antigen. *Am J Med Sci* 263:27-33, 1972.

29. Barker LF, Murray R: Acquisition of hepatitis-associated antigen: Clinical features in young adults. *JAMA* 216:1970-1976, 1971.

30. Haugen RK: Hepatitis after the transfusion of frozen red cells and washed red cells. *N Engl J Med* 301:393-395, 1979.

31. Valeri CR, Zaroulis CG, Vecchione JJ, et al.: Therapeutic effectiveness and safety of outdated human red blood cells rejuvenated to improve oxygen transport function, frozen for about 1½ years at —80 C, washed, and stored at 4 C for 24 hours prior to rapid infusion. *Transfusion,* 20:159-170, 1980.

32. International Forum: What is the clinical importance of alterations in hemoglobin oxygen affinity in preserved blood—especially as produced by variations of red cell 2,3-DPG content? *Vox Sang* 34:111-127, 1978.

33. Metheny D: Clinical estimation of acute blood loss by the Tilt test. *Amer Surg* 33:573-574, 1967.

34. Collins JA: Massive blood transfusion. *Clin Haematol* 5:201-222, 1976.

35. Adamson J, Hillman RS: Blood volume and plasma protein replacement following acute blood loss in normal man. *JAMA* 205:609-612, 1968.

36. Hillman RS (ed): Blood Component Therapy. *Self-Learning Series*. Philadelphia, American College of Physicians, 1977.

37. Shires TD, Coln D, Carrico J, et al: Fluid therapy in hemorrhagic shock. *Arch Surg* 88:688-693, 1964.

38. Gollub S, Bailey CP: Management of major surgical blood loss without transfusion. *JAMA* 198:1171-1174, 1966.

39. Pruitt BA, Moncrief JA, Mason AD: Efficacy of buffered saline as the sole replacement fluid following acute measured hemorrhage in man. *J Trauma* 7:767-782, 1967.

40. Moss GS, Saletta JD: Traumatic shock in man. *N Engl J Med* 290:724-726, 1974.

41. Carey LC, Lowery BD, Cloutier CT: Hemorrhagic shock. *Current Problems in Surgery,* January, 1971.

42. Collins JA: The causes of progressive pulmonary insufficiency in surgical patients. *J Surg Res* 9:685-704, 1969.

43. Alexander B, Odake K, Lawlor D, et al: Coagulation, hemostatis, and plasma expanders: A quarter century enigma. *Fed Proc* 34:1429-1440, 1975.

44. Weil MH: Principles of fluid challenge for routine treatment of shock, in Weil MH, DaLuz PL (eds): *Critical Care Medicine Manual.* New York, Springer-Verlag, 1978, pp 121-128.

45. Bryan-Brown CW: Tissue blood flow and oxygen transport in critically ill patients, in Weil MH, DaLuz PL (eds): *Critical Care Medicine Manual.* New York, Springer-Verlag, 1978, pp 247-257.

46. Linman JW: Physiologic and pathophysiologic effects of anemia. *N Engl J Med* 279:812-818, 1968.

47. Varat MA, Adolph RJ, Fowler NO: Cardiovascular effects of anemia. *Am Heart J* 83:415-426, 1972.

48. Woodson RD, Wills RE, Lenfant C: Effect of acute and established anemia at rest, submaximal and maximal work. *J Applied Physiol* 44:36-43, 1978.

49. Lostumbo MM, Holland PV, Schmidt PJ: Isoimmunization after multiple transfusions. *N Engl J Med* 275:141-144, 1966.

50. Wallerstein RO: Intravenous iron-dextran complex. *Blood* 32:690-695, 1968.

51. Cutting HO, Marlow AA: Partial exchange transfusion in severe chronic anemia. *Arch Intern Med* 117:478-479, 1966.

52. Pearson HA, O'Brien RT: The management of thalassemia major. *Sem Hematol* 12:255-265, 1975.

53. Propper RD, Cooper B, Rufo RR, et al: Continuous subcutaneous administration of deferoxamine in patients with iron overload. *N Engl J Med* 297:418-423, 1977.

Chapter 5

SELECTION OF BLOOD:
COMPATIBILITY DECISIONS

Clareyse Nelson, MT(ASCP)SBB

Introduction

B LOOD compatibility and selection are essential aspects of transfusion therapy. Carefully performed serological testing and other pretransfusion tests can help to ensure that tranfused components have a reasonable physiologic survival and that hemolytic transfusion reactions do not occur. Careful identification of the recipient and donor samples are crucial elements in providing safe transfusion. (See Chapter 2 for guidelines which ensure safe recipient identification and sample collection.)

Pretransfusion Testing

Pretransfusion testing of the recipient sample includes determination of the ABO and Rh groups, performance of an antibody detection test to determine whether unexpected alloantibodies are present in the recipient's serum, and performance of a compatibility test, or crossmatch, between the patient's and donor's blood samples. Identification of any detected antibody should be attempted before blood is provided to the patient. Results of pretransfusion tests should be compared with transfusion service records for blood type and unexpected red cell antibodies that may have been previously identified in the recipient.

Selection of Blood

Selection of blood for compatibility testing is based on the recipient's ABO and Rh groups and on the presence or absence of alloantibodies.[2]

ABO Group

Recipients of blood products containing red cells should receive ABO-specific blood. When ABO-specific blood is not available for a patient, red cells of an ABO group compatible with the recipient's serum can be transfused safely. Guidelines for the selection of the appropriate ABO group are illustrated in Table 1.

41

Table 1.—Selection of Blood According to ABO Type

Patient Type	Donor Type		
	1st choice	2nd choice	3rd choice
O	O	none	
A	A	O red cells	
A_1 with anti-H	A_1	none	
A_2 with anti-A_1	A_2	O red cells	
B	B	O red cells	
AB	AB	A or B* red cells	O red cells
A_1B with anti-H	A_1B	A_1 or B* red cells	
A_2B with anti-A_1	A_2B	A_2 or B* red cells	O red cells

* Either type may be chosen. However, only one of the two should be given to a particular recipient. Usually type A is more readily available and, therefore, is more commonly selected.

When transfusing a patient with ABO-compatible, but not ABO-specific blood, red blood cells should be used rather than whole blood. The plasma in the whole blood contains anti-A or anti-B or both, depending on the blood group. These antibodies will react with the red cell antigens of recipients with other blood groups, particularly when multiple units of O blood are transfused into non-group O recipients. If the antibodies are of low titer and lack hemolytic activity, the risk of recipient red cell destruction is minimal. However, in some donors with high-titer hemolytic activity, the potential risk of recipient red cell hemolysis is greater. This risk can be minimized by removing the plasma, which contains the antibody.

Once blood of a different ABO group is transfused, and ABO-group specific blood becomes available, a decision must be made about changing back to the recipient's blood type. The decision should be based on the following: If a freshly drawn sample of the recipient's serum has circulating anti-A or anti-B antibody, then transfusion of non-ABO-specific blood, compatible with this antibody, should be continued. However, if passively transfused A or B antibody is not detected, it is safe to transfuse the patient with ABO-specific blood.[2]

Blood selection based on specific subgroups of A is not necessary unless the patient has an anti-A_1 or anti-H antibody.[2] In patients with an anti-A_1, either A_2 or A_2B red cells can be transfused. A_1 or A_1B blood would be acceptable for patients with anti-H.

Rh Group

D-positive recipients may receive either D-positive or D-negative blood. It is not essential for known D^u-positive patients to receive Rh-negative blood. Although D^u patients can form anti-D if transfused with D-positive blood, they do so very rarely, and, for all practical purposes, can be considered Rh-positive when selecting blood for transfusion.[3 (p293),4]

Because the D antigen is highly immunogenic, D,D^u-negative red cell products should be tranfused to the D,D^u-negative recipient except under reasonable and qualifying circumstances. Reports show that at least 50% of D-negative recipients will develop anti-D after only a single transfusion of D-positive blood.[3 (p285)] However, in a situation where blood is urgently required for a D-negative recipient and D-negative blood is not available, D-positive crossmatch-compatible blood may be transfused safely to the non-sensitized D-negative recipient. While a patient may subsequently develop anti-D in such cases, transfusion of Rh-positive blood to an Rh-negative individual will not cause a hemolytic transfusion reaction. The worst that could happen is that a sensitized individual would then require only D-negative blood for subsequent transfusions. Consultation between the transfusion service physician and the requesting physician should occur when the decision to transfuse Rh-positive blood to an Rh-negative individual is made.

The selection of blood matched for Rh antigens other than D is not necessary unless the patient has an alloantibody to a particular Rh antigen. D-negative blood that is C- or E-positive can be given to an Rh-negative recipient with little risk of immunization.[4]

Presence of Alloantibodies

When a clinically significant unexpected blood group antibody is detected in a recipient, the antibody should be identified, and donor blood lacking the antigen to which the patient is immunized should be selected for transfusion.

Exceptions may be necessary when blood is urgently needed or if there is insufficient time to identify the antibody. Under these conditions, the transfusion service physician and the patient's physician should both be consulted about the advisability of transfusion.

Compatibility Testing

The final step in pretransfusion testing is determining compatibility between the donor red cells and recipient serum, referred to as "major crossmatch." This test is designed to detect clinically significant red cell antibodies in the recipient directed against antigens on the donor red cells, which would ultimately lead to a transfusion reaction or premature destruction of transfused cells. The crossmatch also detects major errors in ABO grouping or in identification of the donor or recipient. The crossmatch does not necessarily ensure normal survival of transfused red cells, nor does it prevent immunization in the recipient, or detect all unexpected red cell antibodies in the recipient's serum.

Compatibility testing between recipient cells and donor serum—or "minor crossmatch"—is not necessary. Even if antibodies are contained in donor plasma, they are diluted during transfusion; the likelihood of the antibodies causing overt red cell destruction in the recipient with the corresponding antigen is indeed very rare.[5]

Unexpected Antibodies in Recipients

Unexpected red cell alloantibodies are usually found in people who, through pregnancy or previous transfusion, have been exposed to foreign red cell antigens. Some people who have had no known red cell stimulus may also form unexpected antibodies and these usually react at low temperatures. All of these unexpected antibodies normally can be detected in pretransfusion testing by discrepancies between ABO cell and serum grouping, by positive antibody detection tests, or by incompatible cross-matches. Properly selected reagent red cells can usually detect 95% or more of clinically significant red cell antibodies in recipients.[2]

In most cases, when an alloantibody is detected, specificity can be determined using standard technics. Blood that lacks the corresponding antigen should be transfused. More difficult problems may result from the presence of multiple alloantibodies or antibodies to high incidence antigens. Some laboratories may lack the skills necessary to identify such specificities; these samples, thus, should be sent to a reference laboratory. Compatible blood can usually be found, at times, with the help of rare donor files. The medical director of the blood transfusion service should confer with the attending physician when such problems become evident. Transfusions normally do not constitute an emergency, thereby allowing adequate time for the resolution of such problems.

Warm Reacting Antibodies

The incidence of red cell alloantibody formation has been reported by several authors. In 1977, Giblett compiled data regarding the incidence of alloantibody formation in transfusion recipients and donors.[5] She found that the number of patients sensitized to blood group antigens has increased during the past 20 years in spite of a marked drop in the incidence of immunization to Rh. Even though most patients receive blood of their own Rh group, many are immunized by other antigens, especially, K, E, c, Fy[a], and Jk[a]. Another study found that, after anti-D and mixtures of Rh antibodies, the antibodies most commonly formed through transfusion or pregnancy were E, Kell, Fy[a], c, and Jk[a].[6]

44

Table 2.—Incidence of Alloantibodies Reacting at 37 C and After Antiglobulin Testing,* University of Minnesota 1975-78

Specificity	Females	Males	Total	% of Total
anti - D	144	17	161	22%
anti - Kel	81	48	129	18%
anti - E	63	42	105	14%
anti - Le^a	66	24	90	12%
anti - C	52	13	65	9%
anti - c	29	8	37	5%
anti - Lu^a	17	18	35	5%
anti - Fy^a	26	8	34	5%
anti - Le^b	15	13	28	4%
anti - Jk^a	10	6	16	2%
anti - Wr^a	9	2	11	1.5%
anti - S	5	2	7	1%
anti - Fy^b	2	2	4	<1%
anti - e	3	1	4	<1%
anti - C^w	3	1	4	<1%
anti - JK^b	3	1	4	<1%
anti - s	2	0	2	<1%
anti - Kp^a	0	1	1	<1%
Total	530	207	737	

* Incidence of antibodies detected per screening test performed was 1:122.

Table 2 details test results performed at the University of Minnesota from 1975 through 1978 regarding the frequency of antibody formation at 37 C and after antiglobulin testing.[6,7] In total, 70% of the antibodies were found in females and 30% in males. Excluding anti-D, the ratio of antibodies found by sex was 66% in females and 33% in males. It is necessary to transfuse antigen-negative, crossmatch-compatible blood to patients in whom these warm reacting alloantibodies are detected.

The antiglobulin test also detects another group of antibodies, which frequently react to a donor's red cells. While considered "nuisance" antibodies, Sd^a, Ve^a, Ge^a, Yk^a, Co^a, Ch^a, and Rg^a are not known to destroy red cells in vivo.[5] Many patients with anti-Sd^a, anti-Chido, anti-Kn^a, and anti-Yk^a have indeed been transfused with red cells containing the corresponding antigens with no signs of hemolytic transfusion reaction.[8,9] There have been conflicting reports, however, regarding transfusion success in patients who developed antibodies to other high incidence antigens. For example, in one report, an individual with anti-Vel received a unit of Vel-positive blood and had no reaction. In a second case, however, a Vel-negative individual received as little as 30 ml Vel-positive blood and had a severe hemolytic transfusion reaction.[9] Similarly conflicting reports have been published on the hemolytic potential of anti-Yt^a.[3 (p339), 8, 10] An "in vivo crossmatch," using ^{51}Chromium labeled donor red cells may be helpful in assessing potential transfusion reactions due to alloantibodies.[8,11] Also, testing of family members, particularly siblings, may be of great value in finding compatible blood for patients who have antibodies to high incidence antigens. Autologous transfusions should also be considered for such patients.

Room Temperature and Cold-Reacting Alloantibodies

One group of antibodies reacts best at 4 C and may even react up to room temperature. This group includes: anti-P_1, anti-A_1, anti-M, anti-N, and anti-H. Mollison states that, based on red cell survival studies, antibodies that agglutinate cells at about 30 C, but are only slightly active at higher temperatures, cause no destruction in vivo.[3 (p475)] These antibodies are not capable of causing a homolytic transfusion reaction if found unreactive in vitro at 37 C. Further, over a 20-year period, during which over one million units of blood were transfused, Giblett did not observe even a single case of hemolysis, in vivo, caused by such antibodies as anti-P_1, anti-A_1, anti-M, anti-N, and anti-Lu^a.

Lewis antibodies are frequently cold-reacting and only a small proportion of anti-Le^a antibodies are capable of severe red cell destruction.[5] However, since about 80% of all donors have Le(a-) blood, it is practical to give Le(a-) blood even to patients whose serum contains anti-Le^a. The less common anti-Le^b antibody is disregarded by Giblett, except in those unusual cases when the antibody reacts at 37 C.[5] In these situations, if Le(a-b-) blood is unavailable, a recommended course of action is to neutralize the Lewis antibody by using Lewis-positive plasma just prior to transfusion.[3 (p512-514)]

In summary, many transfusion experts feel that clinical hemolysis will not be caused by antibodies that are only detectable at room temperature in vitro. Therefore, room temperature antibody detection and cross-matching probably are not necessary. Some experts, however, are continuing to perform room temperature testing. Either way, if antibody activity is evident at 37 C or after antiglobulin testing, blood that lacks the corresponding antigen should be selected for transfusion.

Cold Autoantibodies

A very common problem encountered in compatibility testing is the presence of naturally occurring cold autoantibodies, notably anti-I or anti-IH, with a titer and thermal amplitude lower than that found in cold agglutinin disease.[12] These antibodies bind complement following the antigen-antibody reaction at low temperatures. After incubation at 37 C and testing with antiglobulin reagents, bound complement may be detected; thus, interfering with the crossmatch test. In this situation, it is important to determine whether there is an underlying clinically significant antibody. One approach to make this determination is to perform the antibody identification procedure and crossmatch test strictly at 37 C.[2,13] If the patient has not been transfused recently, an alternate approach is to perform cold autoabsorption to remove the autoantibody; any underlying clinically significant alloantibodies can thus be detected.[2,13]

Unexpected Antibodies in Donors

The significance of antibodies in donor blood has been exaggerated in the past. Indeed, hemolytic reaction is caused rarely, if ever, by an incompatible antibody (other than anti-A or anti-B) present in the donor's plasma.[3(p 533)] Even anti-A antibodies, which are by far the most destructive of all blood group antibodies, do not ordinarily cause disastrous results when transfused in small amounts to a type-A individual. It is common practice in many hospitals to transfuse plasma-suspended type-O platelets into non-O recipients; only a few patients have demonstrated mild hemolysis. There is no available evidence, which suggests that other naturally occurring antibodies (such as, anti-A_1, anti-P, anti-Le[a], anti-Le[b], anti-M, and anti-N) are potentially destructive when present in donor blood. Laboratory procedures designed to detect these antibodies in donor units should, therefore, be discouraged.[5]

Anti-D is among the alloantibodies most commonly found in donor blood. When present in Rh-negative blood, anti-D does carry a small risk if given to Rh-positive patients, especially if given to infants with hemolytic disease of the newborn. Anti-D carries yet another risk when given to Rh-negative women who are then tested for Rh antibodies before receiving Rh immune globulin. The donor's anti-D might be misinterpreted as the product of the patient's immune system.[5]

Other than anti-D, the incidence of red cell alloantibodies is only about one out of every 1,000 donors.[5] In most cases, the titer of these infrequently occurring antibodies is low. Thus, if a red cell alloantibody is found in donor blood, the unit should not be discarded. If physicians are reluctant to utilize the unit as whole blood, the red cells may be given as packed, washed, or frozen cells.

Emergency Selection of Blood

The most important aspect of the immediate care of a patient who has lost a large volume of blood is maintenance of the patient's blood volume. Therapy should be initiated at once by using colloid (ie, plasma protein, fraction, albumin, plasma, hydroxyethyl starch, or dextran) and electrolyte solutions. There is no advantage to using whole blood or red cells to maintain blood volume. In fact, with limited or no crossmatch, whole blood and red cells will increase the risk of hemolytic transfusion reaction.

After crossmatching procedures have been carried out, blood should be selected after clinically assessing its risks against the urgency of its need. Several criteria for emergency blood selection are listed below.

Uncrossmatched Group-O, Rh-Negative Red Blood Cells

Group-O, Rh-negative red blood cells with the plasma removed may be utilized in cases of extreme emergency when there is not enough time to determine the patient's blood group. However, a blood sample should be collected immediately prior to transfusion. Blood grouping and compatibility testing should be performed on all blood units even though the transfusion has already been initiated.[1]

Uncrossmatched ABO and Rh-Specific Blood

ABO and Rh blood grouping can be carried out within minutes and group-specific blood can be issued. Blood transfusion services supporting emergency rooms should be organized in such a way that grouping can be done at once, thereby, reducing the need to use group-O, Rh-negative red cells. In fact, with immediate blood grouping, it is very rare to require more than one unit of group-O Rh-negative red cells. But if the unit is required, standard compatibility tests should be completed promptly.

Abbreviated Crossmatch

An abbreviated crossmatch and antibody screening test can be performed in an emergency situation. Blood can be issued after an immediate spin crossmatch. Alternatively, a shortened incubation time can be utilized for the compatibility test.

Transfusion reactions may occur if the patient has unexpected antibodies to red cell antigens. The relative risks of the shortened crossmatch depend on whether the patient has been previously screened for unexpected red cell antibodies, which may cause a hemolytic transfusion reaction. If previous screens detected no unexpected clinically significant antibodies, and blood has been run through an immediate spin crossmatch, it can be considered relatively risk free.[14]

This procedure is riskier in the patient who has never been screened for antibodies. The risk is minimal in the patient who has never been transfused nor has ever been pregnant, and increases in relation to the number of previous transfusions and pregnancies. In a patient population studied at the Puget Sound Blood Center in 1974 and 1975, 1.6% had unexpected antibodies (excluding Lewis antibodies).[5] A crossmatch using a shortened incubation time and an antiglobulin test can minimize the risk in the patient who has never been screened for antibodies by detecting all but the weakest blood group antibodies. In one report, 97% of serums containing blood group antibodies gave a positive reaction after 15 minutes of incubation and performing the antiglobulin test.[3(p 441)]

An emergency situation may arise in which a patient needing blood has known red cell alloantibodies that react only after performing an antiglobulin crossmatch. If there is no time to do the test, immediate consultation between the transfusion service medical director and the patients's physician is required.

Surgical Blood Orders

Because of the relatively short shelf life (21 days) of blood, it is important that transfusion service medical directors and other physicians can carefully manage blood inventory. One approach is to increase the availability of blood resources. Another approach is to utilize blood resources effectively. Appropriate crossmatch ordering is an important factor in achieving proper utilization. Crossmatched blood is usually reserved for a particular patient from 24 to 48 hours, and is thus withheld for use in other patients. The blood often becomes outdated if it is not transfused to the patient for whom it was originally crossmatched. By reducing the amount of time each unit spends in an assigned or crossmatched status, outdating can be curtailed and more blood will become available for transfusion.

Several authors have demonstrated that elective surgery is an area in which excessive crossmatching may occur.[15-19] Therefore, by establishing preoperative crossmatch guidelines resulting in standard blood orders for elective surgical procedures, hospital transfusion services can manage blood inventory more effectively.

Type and Screen

Standard surgical blood orders include a "type and screen"—ABO and Rh grouping and screening for unexpected antibodies—on patients prior to elective surgical procedures that rarely require hemotherapy (eg, cholecystectomy, hemorrhoidectomy, D&C, gastrostomy, or appendectomy).

When "type and screen" is being used, the transfusion service must consider several factors. First, these patients do require blood, although rarely, and it may be necessary to transfuse blood with only a partial

49

crossmatch. It is very important that the antibody screening procedure is carefully designed and meticulously carried out so that clinically significant antibodies can be detected and identified. Blood lacking the corresponding antigen should be made available for the operative procedure.

Even when the screening test is negative, blood of compatible ABO and Rh groups should be available, on demand, from the transfusion service inventory. The communication between the operating room and transfusion service must be swift and efficient so that blood can be provided immediately, when it is needed.

If blood is needed, a crossmatch can be completed in less than an hour. In an emergency, a transfusion can be initiated before a crossmatch is complete. Previous grouping and antibody screening of the patient's blood ensures that a transfusion will be 99.9% safe.[7] In a retrospective study of 82,647 crossmatches performed on 13,950 patients who had negative antibody screening tests, only eight incompatible crossmatches, reacting after the immediate spin phase of the crossmatch, were related to antibodies that would be considered clinically significant.[14] Therefore, blood issued after the "immediate spin" phase of the crossmatch to a patient with a previous negative antibody screen, may be transfused with a very low level of risk. Every case should be considered individually, so that it may be advisable to crossmatch blood for those patients who are anemic or have coagulation problems.

Standard Surgical Blood Orders

In addition to the "type and screen," a standard surgical blood order can be implemented. A predetermined number of blood units are crossmatched for those patients who are likely to need transfusions during elective surgery. Blood order guidelines should be based on previous transfusion requirements for common elective surgical procedures in a particular institution. The purpose of the guidelines is to provide an appropriate amount of crossmatched blood that will be available for elective surgery patients.

Several authors have published blood order guidelines established by their own institutions. Table 3 compares guidelines of several large blood transfusion services and includes data on the number of transfusions required during elective surgery procedures in these institutions.

Successful implementation of a standard surgical blood order schedule requires close cooperation between the transfusion service medical director and the surgical and anesthesiology staff. They should all agree on preoperative blood orders for particular procedures in advance. Further, a mechanism for modifying the orders according to individual patients' needs should be made available. For example, additional precautions may

50

Table 3.—Suggested Surgical Blood Orders for Elective Surgical Procedures: A Comparison of Four Institutions

Procedure	State University of New York Upstate Medical Center	Los Angeles County/ University of Southern California Medical Center	University of Michigan	University of Minnesota
General Surgery				
Cholecystectomy	T + S*	T + S	0-1	T + S → 1
Cholectomy	2	2	3	2
Cholostomy (closure, revision)	T + S	T + S	1	
Exploratory laparotomy	T + S	2	2	1-3
Gastrectomy	3	2	2	2
Hernia repair	T + S	T + S	0-2	T + S
Mastectomy-radical	1	2	2	1
Splenectomy	1	T + S		2
Thoroacotomy (biopsy)	2	T + S		1-3
Thyroidectomy	T + S	T + S	T + S	T + S → 1
Vagotomy & pyloroplasty		T + S		1
Vascular Surgery				
Aortic aneurism repair	6	2	4 → 5	7
Carotid endarterectomy	1	T + S	2	1 → 2
Heart revascularization	8	2	8 → 9	9
Valve replacement				
Aortic	8	4		9
Mitral	8	2		9
Neuro Surgery				
Craniotomy	2	T + S		2
aneurism	4 → 6	2	6	
Laminectomy (disc)	0	T + S	2	1
Obstetrics/Gynecology				
Caesarean section		T + S	1 → 2	1
D & C	T + S	T + S	0 → 1	0
Hysterectomy:				
Total abdominal	T + S	T + S	2	3
Vaginal	T + S	T + S	2	
Radical	4	4	3	
Laparoscopic tubal ligation	T + S	T + S	T + S	T + S
Orthopedic Surgery				
Amputation (AK or BK)	T + S	T + S	1	1
Arthrotomy	T + S	T + S	T + S	T + S
Hip: nailing	2	4	2	2
replacement	5	4	5 → 6	4
Open reduction-extremities	1	T + S → 4		3

Continued.

	Otorhinolaryngology			
Laryngectomy	2		4	
Maxillectomy	2		6	4
Parotidectomy	T + S		2	
Radical neck dissection	2		4	2 → 4
T & A			T + S	0
	Urology			
Cystectomy-radical	4		4	6
Nephrectomy	2	2	2	2
Orchiectomy	T + S		T + S	T + S
Prostatectomy	2-3		2	4
Pyelolithotomy	T + S	T + S		1
Trans-urethral resection: prostrate	T + S	T + S	2	1

* Type and screen

be necessary in patients with anemia or bleeding disorders. A surgeon must be confident in the ability of his transfusion service to provide blood rapidly in times of emergency; therefore, a mechanism for rapidly and effectively providing blood should be established. Finally, it is recommended that each hospital develop its own crossmatch guidelines based on its own surgical experience. This will ensure that variations in surgical technic and expertise will be reflected. Coordination of policy by the Transfusion Committee may be helpful.

In summary, the implementation of preoperative surgical guidelines can result in reduced and realistic crossmatch ordering, and thus lead to savings in transfusion service work load, patient charges, and blood utilization.

References

1. *Standards for Blood Banks and Transfusion Services,* ed 9. Washington, DC, American Association of Blood Banks, 1978.
2. *Technical Manual.* Washington, DC, American Association of Blood Banks, 1977, pp 188-198.
3. Mollison PL: *Blood Transfusion in Clinical Medicine,* ed 5. London, Blackwell Scientific Publications, 1972.
4. Huestis DW, Bove JR, Busch S: *Practical Blood Transfusion,* ed 2. Boston, Little, Brown and Co, 1976, p 210.
5. Giblett ER: Blood group alloantibodies: An assessment of some laboratory practices. *Transfusion* 17:299-308, 1977.
6. Spielmann W, Seidl S: Prevalence of irregular red cell antibodies and their significance in blood transfusion and antenatal care. *Vox Sang* 26: 551-559, 1974.

7. Boral LI, Henry JB: The type and screen: A safe alternative and supplement in selected surgical procedures. *Transfusion* 17:163-168, 1977.
8. Silvergleid AJ, Wells RF, Hafleigh EB, et al: Compatibility testing using [51]Chromium-labelled red blood cells in crossmatch positive patients. *Transfusion* 18:8-14, 1978.
9. Moulds JJ: Multiple and high-incidence antibodies, in *Transfusion With "Crossmatch-Incompatible" Blood*. Washington, DC, American Association of Blood Banks, 1975, pp 47-53.
10. Bettigole R, Harris JP, Tegoli J, et al: Rapid in vivo destruction of Yt(a+) red cells in a patient with anti Yt[a]. *Vox Sang* 14:143, 1968.
11. Bell CA, Stroup M: Autoimmune problems, in *Transfusion With "Crossmatch Incompatible" Blood*. Washington, DC, American Association of Blood Banks, 1975, pp 12-14.
12. Garratty G, Petz LD, Hoops J: The correlation of cold agglutinin titrations in saline and albumin with haemolytic anemia. *Br J Haematol* 35:587, 1977.
13. Nichols ME: Cold autoantibodies and alloantibodies, in *Trouble-Shooting the Crossmatch*. Washington, DC, American Association of Blood Banks, 1977, pp 27-29.
14. Oberman HA, Barnes BA, Friedman BA: The risk of abbreviating the major crossmatch in urgent or massive transfusion. *Transfusion* 18:137-141, 1978.
15. Friedman BA, Oberman HA, Chadwick AR, et al: The maximum surgical blood order schedule and surgical blood use in the United States. *Transfusion* 16:380-387, 1976.
16. Mintz PD, Nordine RB, Henry JB, et al: Expected hemotherapy in elective surgery. *NY State J Med* 76:532-537, 1976.
17. ———, Lauenstein K, Hume J, et al: Expected hemotherapy in elective surgery, a follow-up. *JAMA* 239: 623-625, 1978.
18. Rouault C, Gruenhagen J: Reorganization of blood ordering practices. *Transfusion* 18:448-453, 1978.
19. Devitt JE: Blood wastage and cholecystectomy: spin-off from a peer review. *Can Med Assoc J* 109:120, 1973.

Chapter 6

MANAGEMENT OF MASSIVE AND EMERGENCY TRANSFUSION

E. Arthur Dreskin, MD

Massive Blood Transfusion

A MASSIVE blood transfusion is commonly regarded as the rapid replacement of one's total blood volume, ie, 10 to 12 units of blood within a 12-hour period.[1] Massive blood transfusions usually are indicated in cases of acute hemorrhage occurring during operative procedures, during treatment of major trauma, and commonly in cardiopulmonary bypass procedures. An exchange transfusion is one form of massive transfusion.

Because of the importance of blood volume replacement and oxygen-carrying function in these procedures, whole blood is commonly administered in massive transfusions. This does not preclude the use of packed cells with supplemental plasma (particularly fresh or fresh frozen plasma), or serum albumin. Frozen red cells are acceptable for massive blood replacement, but should be given with plasma protein fraction or fresh frozen plasma.

Rapid infusion of large amounts of blood can be achieved by: 1) administration under pressure; or 2) using multiple infusion sites to simultaneously administer several units. Rapid infusion is also facilitated by using a larger-than-customary-size needle, ie, 15 or 16 gauge, or by inserting a plastic catheter into the vein. When necessary, a complete unit of blood may be administered in less than five minutes. There have been cases where as many as 50 to 100 units of blood have been administered within a 24-hour period.[2] Massive transfusions may involve problems not ordinarily encountered in routine blood administration. Several such problems will be discussed in detail.

Hemostasis

The patient receiving large quantities of blood may ooze from cut surfaces and may even continue bleeding postoperatively. This is due, in part, to dilution of coagulation factors, to consumption and the resulting quantitative loss of such coagulation factors as V, VIII, and IX, and to a decrease in platelets ("platelet washout"). Deficiencies in coagulation factors can be best treated with fresh frozen plasma. Loss of platelets to low levels may require platelet transfusion. These abnormalities often improve spontaneously as the clinical state of the patient improves. Recent studies have shown that hypotension, due to massive blood loss, may in itself contribute to poor hemostasis.[3]

Recent studies indicate that CPD blood may retain coagulation factors (such as Factor V and VIII) significantly better than ACD blood. This is important because older studies demonstrating a reduction in the coagulation factors in stored blood used ACD-anticoagulated blood, which is rarely used today.

One unit of whole blood less than five days old or fresh frozen plasma (FFP) with packed cells is often given routinely after five to ten units of stored blood have been administered. [1,4] If further transfusion is needed, this protocol is followed with each additional five units of stored blood. The need for the addition of coagulation factors has been questioned and is discussed at length in Chapter 12. In massive transfusion cases platelet deficiencies are usually relatively mild and normally, patients receiving massive amounts of blood will recover spontaneously from thrombocytopenia and will not bleed. In patients where thrombocytopenia is shown to be a factor in bleeding, the administration of platelet concentrates is indicated. The number of units given depends on the initial platelet level of the patient and the platelet increment desired (see Chapter 9). A platelet count over 50,000 per cu mm should be maintained in the presence of open wounds or when critical organs are exposed.

Recent studies of coagulation changes in massively transfused patients indicate that disseminated intravascular coagulation (DIC) may be an important causal factor in bleeding following the use of stored blood in large quantities. The relationship between DIC and bleeding may be due to thromboplastic substances in stored blood; to a superimposed abnormality of consumption; or to an occult transfusion reaction which is, in itself, a powerful stimulant to the formation of a consumption coagulopathy. DIC, however, is usually due to the underlying disease process. Treatment for suspected DIC should be directed primarily toward the underlying disease and would be supportive in nature. Fresh frozen plasma and platelets are indicated in treating some cases of DIC. The administration of heparin is often advised, even though its efficacy in treating DIC is not conclusive.

Temperature of Blood

Hypothermia can result from rapid administration of large volumes of cold blood. The incidence of cardiac arrest has been shown to be increased in severely ill patients receiving large amounts of cold blood.

It has also been demonstrated that warming blood will reduce the risks of cardiac complications in massive transfusion.[6] It is, therefore, common practice to use warmed blood when over five units of blood must be administered rapidly. The blood warmer must be designed to warm large quantities of blood to 32 C, even when large quantities of blood are given rapidly. (See Chapter 3 for an in-depth discussion on blood warmers.)

Microaggregates

It is a standard practice to administer all blood through a filter to remove such material as aggregated platelets, fibrin clots, and cellular debris. The commonly used transfusion filter set has a 170μ pore size. Recently, several filters have been developed that have a pore size as small as 20μ. These filters can remove particulate matter that would normally pass through a standard filter, thus causing microemboli.[7,8] (See Chapter 3, section on Microaggregate Filters.) The standard 170μ filters suffice for frozen or recently centrifuged packed red blood cells, since processing frozen blood removes microaggregates and "packing" centrifuged cells removes or increases the size of the microparticles.

Acid-Base Studies

Older studies of acid-base balance following massive transfusion were based on the use of ACD blood, which appreciably enhanced acid levels, as a result of citric acid, present in the anticoagulant, and lactic acid, generated during storage. Both are rapidly metabolized under normal conditions. Patients requiring massive transfusions usually are also in a state of metabolic acidosis, which rapidly reverses when blood volume is restored by adequate tissue perfusion. The final success of blood transfusion depends on a complex interaction of blood volume, the rate of metabolic change and the circulatory status of the recipient. Collins studied a group of massively transfused Viet Nam casualties and found that controlling hemorrhage and blood pressure were the most important factors in the regulation of infused acid load and pre-existant metabolic acidosis.[9] An important conclusion of the study was that exogenous alkalinization was of no benefit to the patients. A routine evaluation of blood gases during massive transfusion procedures should determine the acid-base status of the patient and the need for specific therapy.

CPD blood, which has a higher, more physiologic pH (7.0 after seven days storage[10]) is in widespread use today. The initial acidemic effect of CPD blood is substantially lower than that of ACD anti-coagulated blood. However, the metabolic alkalosis that ultimately occurs with CPD blood may increase hemoglobin's affinity for oxygen, thereby, retarding the release of oxygen to the tissues.

Hemoglobin Function

Hemoglobin's affinity for oxygen is influenced considerably by the concentration of 2,3-diphosphoglyceric acid (2,3-DPG).[11] 2,3-DPG is maintained at near normal levels for seven days in stored CPD blood, decreasing to a 50% level at 14 days. A depletion of this enzyme increases hemoglobin's affinity for oxygen, and makes hemoglobin inefficient in delivering oxygen to peripheral tissues. Thus, the patient who receives a massive transfusion of older stored blood may produce a hemoglobin-oxygen affinity shift in a direction opposite to that which is desirable; therefore, tissues may be deprived of needed oxygen. 2,3-DPG will, however, regenerate rapidly following transfusion and reaches a normal level within 24 hours. The acid-base status (acidosis) of the patient may concomitantly and adversely influence the rate of 2,3-DPG regeneration. Hypothermia[5] also affects the release of oxygen to the tissues, increasing hemoglobin's affinity for oxygen.

Thus, it is desirable to use relatively fresh, warmed blood for massive transfusions. CPD blood less than one week old supplies 2,3-DPG in adequate amounts and does not, in itself, affect the acid-base status of the patient. Fresh-frozen or rejuvenated red cells have a normal level of 2,3-DPG and can be used in transfusion situations requiring immediate hemoglobin function. This is particularly important in infant blood exchange transfusions.

Citrate Toxicity

The concept of citrate toxicity has been associated with massive blood replacement for a long time. There is concern both with the citrate level in the blood, which may produce hypotension, and the chemical binding of calcium by citrate, which can lead to tetany and cardiac arrest.[12] The citrate is metabolized by cells throughout the body and is particularly metabolized by the liver. Normally, citrate is removed rapidly. Accumulation of a toxic level of citrate is often caused by very rapid administration of blood in large quantities or by impaired liver function, and is commonly seen in infants during exchange transfusion. In these patients, the citrate level can become critical. Procedures for managing citrate levels are relatively simple: stopping or slowing down the transfusion reduces the citrate concentration in blood and is usually all that is necessary to avoid toxicity. If the blood is administered to adults at a rate not exceeding one unit every five minutes, the transfusion citrate can usually be handled by the body.[13]

Clotting deficiency due to binding of calcium has not been documented in blood transfusions. Patients, in whom a high plasma citrate is likely (leading to hypocalcemia), can be given ionizable calcium, eg, calcium chloride, or calcium gluconate, 10 ml of a 10% solution. It has been customary to give calcium in this dosage with every 10 units of blood administered during a massive transfusion. However, recent evidence has shown that the administration of calcium in high doses can produce an iatrogenic hypercalcemia, which may be more harmful to the patient than helpful.[14] Howland stated that the administration of calcium salts appears unnecessary during massive transfusion and might be harmful, even if given in therapeutic amounts.[15] Mollison's assertion that a warm adult with a functioning liver can tolerate a unit of blood every five minutes without requiring supplemental calcium appears to be a useful rule to follow.[13] It may be helpful to use the calcium ion electrode to follow the serum level of ionized calcium in these patients.[16] Calcium therapy could then be carried out on a more scientific basis. The normal ionized calcium level ranges from 4.0 to 4.8 mgm/dl. Symptomatic hypocalcemia occurs when the ionized calcium level falls below 2.5 mgm/dl but even at these levels Howland did not find significant cardiovascular changes.

Potassium Levels

Stored blood that is more than two weeks old contains a significant level of potassium that is released from the still viable red cells into the plasma. Despite this increase in potassium, hyperkalemia has not been proven as a problem in massive transfusions in adults. Following transfusion, the red cells rapidly absorb potassium and correct any potassium imbalance in the circulation.[17] Collins recently expressed concern about the relation of high potassium and low ionized calcium.[18] On the other hand, Howland, in the same symposium[19] stated that he did not consider hyperkalemia to be either a real or theoretic problem.

Plasticiser Toxicity

Plasticisers, such as diethylhydroxyphthallate (DEHP), used in vinyl plastic blood bags are fat-soluble and leach into the blood during storage.[20] A significant amount of foreign material may be transfused by the time multiple units of blood are given. While current evidence indicates that the plasticisers are well tolerated if infused into adults, toxic and even lethal effects on the embryos of experimental animals have been demonstrated.[21] Thus, the significance of plasticisers in massive transfusions is not clear. Clinically it does not appear to represent a hazard.[5]

59

Phosphate and Ammonia Levels

Phosphate and ammonia levels may become significantly elevated during prolonged storage of blood. In cases of decreased liver function with impending coma, blood that is less than seven days old should be used. Ammonia accumulation in older stored blood may lead to possible ill effects. The use of packed red cells with fresh or fresh frozen plasma is equally, if not more, effective because the potential for increased ammonia is removed. Also, the provision of clotting factors in the frozen plasma is potentially of great significance in liver failure. Preparation of packed cells just prior to transfusion removes the maximum amount of ammonia. The increased phosphate level of stored blood, even with CPD blood, does not represent a known problem.

Hazards of Transfusion

Because of the many units of blood used during a massive transfusion, the risk of disease transmission, particularly hepatitis transmission, is increased. Hepatitis testing can significantly reduce, but cannot eliminate transmission. Emergency blood demand also increases the potential for clerical error. Incompatibility between donors may pose a risk but testing is not necessary on a routine basis and incompatibility problems may be more theoretical than real. Wilson et al point out the infrequency of such reactions in massively transfused patients: Out of a recorded 625 reactions (0.7% of 8529 units given), donor incompatibility was the cause in only 35 cases.[3]

Summary

Several guidelines for the proper transfusion of massive amounts of blood have been outlined in this chapter. CPD anticoagulant is considered superior for use in massive transfusions. The use of blood less than 10 to 14 days old, or red cells centrifuged just prior to use, will prevent the accumulation of chemical substances, which may be present in older blood. Packed red cells with fresh or fresh-frozen plasma provide coagulation factors and can minimize many difficulties. Platelet concentrates are available in modern transfusion services and can be used, as indicated, in platelet-deficient patients. The administration of blood at a physiological temperature will prevent hypothermia and its complications. Where oxygen-carrying capacity is concerned, CPD-stored red cells, 10 days old or less, are superior. Freshly frozen or rejuvenated red cells provide a normal level of 2,3-DPG, thereby permitting normal oxygen release. Considering the often critical status of massively transfused patients, the use of blood as a therapeutic modality is generally quite benign and the alternatives considerably more risky.

References

1. *Technical Manual,* ed 7. Washington, DC, American Association of Blood Banks, 1977, p 191.
2. Kiel F: Development of a blood program in Viet Nam. *Milit Med* 131:1469-1482, 1966.
3. Wilson RF, Mammen E, Walt AJ: Eight years of experience with massive transfusions. *J Trauma* 2:275-285, 1971.
4. Gill W, Chapion HR, Long WB, et al: Volume resuscitation in critical major trauma. *J R Coll Surg Edinb* 20:166-173, 1975.
5. Collins JA: Massive blood transfusion. *Clin Haematol* 5:210-222, 1976.
6. Boyan DP: Cold or warmed blood for massive transfusions. *Ann Surg* 160: 282-286, 1964.
7. Reul GT, Greensburg SD, Lefrale EA: Prevention of postraumatic pulmonary insufficiency: Fine screen filtering of blood. *Arch Surg* 106:386-394, 1973.
8. Solis RT, Gibbs MB: Filtration of the microaggregates in stored blood. *Transfusion* 12:245-250, 1972.
9. Collins JA: Problems associated with the massive transfusion of stored blood. *Surgery* 75:274-295, 1974.
10. Gibson VG, Gregory CB, Butler LN: Citrate-phosphate-dextrose solution for preservation of human blood. *Transfusion* 1:380-387, 1961.
11. Bunn HF, Moy MM, Kocholaty WF, et al: Hemoglobin function of stored blood. *J Clin Invest* 48:311-321, 1969.
12. Bunker JP, Stetson JB, Coe RC, et al: Citric acid intoxication. *JAMA* 157:1361-1367, 1955.
13. Mollison PL: *Blood Transfusion in Clinical Medicine,* ed 5. Oxford, Blackwell Scientific Publications, 1975.
14. Wolf PL, McCarthy LJ, Hafleigh B: Extreme hypercalcemia following blood transfusions combined with intravenous calcium. *Vox Sang* 19:544-545, 1977.
15. Howland WS, Schweizer O, Carlon GC, et al: The cardiovascular effects of low levels of ionized calcium during massive transfusion. *Surg Gynecol Obstet* 145:581-586, 1977.
16. Sorell M, Rosen JF: Ionized calcium-serum levels during symptomatic hypocalcemia. *J Pediatr* 87: 67-70, 1975.
17. Valeri CR: Viability and function of preserved red cells. *N Engl J Med* 284:81-88, 1971.
18. Collins JA: Massive Transfusion: What is Current and Important?, in *Massive Transfusion.* Washington, DC, American Association of Blood Banks, 1978, pp 1-16.

19. Howland WS: Calcium, potassium and pH changes during massive transfusion, in *Massive Transfusion*. Washington, DC, American Association of Blood Banks, 1978, pp 17-24.
20. Marcel YL, Noel SP: Contamination of blood stored in plastic packs. *Lancet* IL35-36, 1970.
21. Roggen G, Bentschmann M, Berchtold H, et al: A contribution to the comparative chemical and biological assay procedures for plastic containers used for blood preservation. *Vox Sang* 9:546-548, 1964.

Chapter 7

AUTOLOGOUS TRANSFUSION

Julian B. Schorr, MD

Introduction

IT MUST HAVE been fairly early in man's history that the dire effects
of severe blood loss were first noted. But it was not until 1818, two
centuries after Harvey described the circulatory system, that John Blundell successfully reinfused vaginal blood salvaged from women with
postpartum bleeding.[1] During the next one hundred years, autologous
transfusion was largely limited to returning blood shed by patients with
hemorrhagic complications of pregnancy.[2, 3, 4]

Late in the nineteenth century, reports describing salvage of shed blood
in other surgical conditions appeared.[5-7] The earliest elective autologous
transfusion was described in 1921.[8] Using 0.2% sodium citrate as the
anticoagulant, Grant drew blood from a man about to undergo surgery
for a brain tumor, stored it overnight, and reinfused it the following day.

The first nonsurgical autologous transfusion was probably performed by
Halsted, who treated a patient with carbon monoxide poisoning by removing, oxygenating, and then reinfusing 500 ml aliquots of his blood.[9]

The historical aspects of autologous transfusion have been extensively
reviewed by Brzica et al[10] and Kuban.[11] Today, autologous transfusion
refers not only to the reinfusion of whole blood previously collected
from the recipient, but to the reinfusion of concentrates of individual
blood components collected and stored for varying periods of time.

Because the types of autologous transfusion differ considerably in
purpose, methodology, advantages and disadvantages, they will be discussed separately.

Intraoperative Autologous Transfusion:
Salvage of Shed Blood

Definition and History

Intraoperative autologous transfusion (IAT) involves the collection,
anticoagulation, filtration and reinfusion of blood which has been shed
during surgery, or as the result of trauma or obstetrical catastrophe.

Early attempts at IAT employed crude instrumentation. Usually, blood
was swabbed from the operative field, the swabs rinsed with saline and

63

the washings reinfused. Burch[12] suggested that if the blood appeared overly contaminated it could be returned via rectal drip. This suggestion never caught fire.

Before the introduction of citrate anticoagulant in 1915[13] a variety of means of preventing extracorporeal clotting were attempted, including defibrination, and the use of ammonium sulfate or phosphate of soda. With current methodology, anticoagulation is achieved by heparinizing the patient, and/or by adding heparin or citrate-phosphate-dextrose (CPD) to the collection reservoir.

In the 1920s, reports on autologous transfusion began to describe aspiration of the shed blood via syringe or suction apparatus.[12, 14] Soon after, hemolysis of the suctioned blood was noted,[15] as was the subsequent development of hemoglobinuria in some patients receiving intraoperative autologous transfusion.[16]

Recent Improvements

The modern era of IAT may be said to have coincided with the development of equipment specifically designed for salvage of shed blood. In 1966, Dyer described a two-chambered glass unit designed to permit gentle aspiration of shed blood without foaming, and to permit its anticoagulation and filtration prior to reinfusion.[17] In 1968, Klebanoff and Watkins introduced the apparatus which, modified somewhat, is now marketed as the Bentley Autotransfusion System ATS 100 (Bentley Laboratories, Irvine, CA).[18]

The ATS 100 consists of a disposable reservoir and attached tubing, through which shed blood is retrieved, anticoagulated and retransfused after defoaming and filtering. The blood is moved in and out of the system by inflow roller pumps.

A number of reports of the successful use of this apparatus have appeared within the last decade.[19-23] In several reports, modifications of the system were used, altering the relatively small capacity of the ATS reservoir, and more importantly eliminating the risk of air embolization, inherent in the Bentley System because blood leaves the reservoir under pressure. As the level in the reservoir falls below a critical point, a photoelectric cell triggers an audible alarm, signaling a dangerous infusion of air. If the signal is interrupted by a clot in the reservoir, or if the warning is ignored or not heard, the patient can be injected with air inadvertently.

Raines et al[23] increased the System's capacity by using two reservoirs; one for collection and one for reinfusion. They also introduced larger roller heads, which they believed would reduce the damage to red blood cells. In addition, they added an anti-air embolus device, through which the reinfusion line passes. This device uses a light-emitting diode, and receiver, which, if it detects as little as 0.25 cm³ air, automatically clamps the line and simultaneously stops the reinfusion roller pump.

Recently, a number of other devices have been developed that salvage blood shed during surgical procedures. The Sorenson Corporation (Salt Lake City, UT) has developed several autotransfusion devices. The most recent model consists of a disposable 1900 ml plastic bag to which varying amounts of CPD are added in a ratio of 7:1. The blood is then reinfused by gravity, using a standard or micropore blood administration filter attached to the outlet spike at the bottom of the bag.[24-26] Other devices for collecting and reinfusing shed blood have been described by Symbas; Welch et al; Johnson et al; and Mattox.[27-30]

Beginning in 1968, with Wilson and Taswell's[31] description of the use of the IBM-NCI continuous flow centrifuge, there has been increasing interest in technics whereby blood is collected during surgical procedures, washed free of debris, supernatant hemoglobin, and cells other than erythrocytes, and then reinfused as washed packed red blood cells.[32] Watson-Williams et al[33] and Moran et al[34] described such a device (Cell Saver, Haemonetics Corporation, Natick, MA), designed to recover autologous blood from the oxygenator following cardiopulmonary bypass surgery. The Cell Saver has also been used to salvage blood shed during other types of surgery.[11,19,35,36]

Complications of Intraoperative Autologous Transfusion

Aside from the danger of air embolization, all of the systems used to aspirate blood from a wound traumatize the patient's erythrocytes and platelets to some extent. A number of studies describe the effect of the salvage technic on blood elements.[19-21,23,26,28,37,38] Although the reported observations are somewhat varied, they all report red cell damage sufficient to cause intravascular hemolysis and hemoglobinemia following retransfusion of unwashed shed blood. It has been suggested that elevated levels of free hemoglobin can accelerate intravascular coagulation, and directly or indirectly cause kidney damage.[39] The use of devices that wash aspirated blood prior to reinfusion almost completely obviates any such possibility.

Thrombocytopenia can be expected following extracorporeal bypass, during which a patient is transfused with blood that has been shed and recovered. The tendency toward thrombocytopenia is enhanced by IAT, where air-blood interface is greater than in cardiopulmonary bypass surgery.[38] Brener and his associates found that platelet metabolism and aggregation are altered during IAT.[40] Duncan et al attributed fatal hemorrhage in three patients to disseminated intravascular coagulopathy (DIC) induced by the autotransfusion apparatus.[41]

65

In addition to the report by Duncan et al,[41] a number of studies on auto-transfused patients have reported changes in coagulation factor levels characteristic of DIC, ie, low levels of Factors I, II, V, VII and VIII, as well as increased levels of fibrin split products.[20,23,27,38] These changes were of brief duration and did not appear to contribute to any increased bleeding tendency. Again, these changes appeared less among patients autotransfused with washed erythrocytes, except in cases of massive transfusions. In general, while autotransfusion can cause DIC, it seems likely that the major contributing factor is the patient's underlying condition, be it shock or significant tissue damage,[10] and not the process of autotransfusion.

Blood removed from a wound may contain debris as well as platelet and leukocyte aggregates. Whether these particles play any role in producing pulmonary insufficiency is conjectural. The potential, if it exists, may be obviated by using a microaggregate filter in the reinfusion line, and can be totally eliminated by using a cell-washing device.

Contraindications

Although collection of blood for autotransfusion in the face of a ruptured gall bladder or a lacerated loop of intestine is probably contraindicated, several reports have suggested that blood that has been grossly contaminated with fecal material may be safely reinfused.[20,22] Glover et al[20] studied 14 patients who were reinfused with shed blood contaminated with fecal material, urine or bile. Seven survived the immediate postoperative period; of these, five had positive blood cultures 24 hours posttransfusion. None of the five developed evidence of sepsis or any other complication that could be related to the autotransfusion.

Autologous transfusion of blood collected during cancer surgery may be contraindicated due to the possibility of spreading malignant cells. In one study, Yaw et al[42] demonstrated that tumor cells were transferred from the operative field to blood aspirated into an autotransfusion device.

Summary

It has become increasingly clear that the reinfusion of salvaged blood can be a valuable adjunct in treating the acutely hemorrhaging patient. The situations most amenable to IAT include traumatic bleeding, and thoracic, gynecologic, vascular, orthopedic and neurologic surgery. Heparinization of patients, other than those undergoing cardiovascular bypass surgery seems on the wane and the most recent reports do not recommend systemic anticoagulation.[20,22,23,25-27] A written protocol should include criteria for the selection of the anticoagulants, and the indicated dosage. If not used immediately, blood collected for IAT should be labeled "For Autologous Transfusion Only" and stored in the usual manner. The expiration date for salvaged blood is 24 hours after its collection. Post-IAT laboratory tests should be performed, as indicated, and usually include an evaluation of hemoglobin level, and of the coagulation status of the patient.

While all of the systems described can successfully salvage shed blood, those which permit reinfusion of a red cell concentrate containing little anticoagulant, which is also free of debris, cellular aggregates and extracellular hemoglobin, appear preferable. Unfortunately, these systems tend to be more complicated and more expensive to operate. However, some institutions consider cell washing devices cost-effective and able to provide the patient with the best form of transfusion and, thus, have begun to utilize the systems on a fairly routine basis.

The major reason that IAT is not accepted for use appears to be that the institution is not willing to provide the equipment and trained staff on a 24-hour-per-day basis. Once this hurdle is overcome, IAT can have a meaningful role both in the emergency suite and the operating room.

Finally, the applicability of IAT to patients who are Jehovah's Witnesses remains moot. Their religious beliefs proscribe the removal, storage and subsequent reinfusion of blood whether that blood is homologous or autologous.[43] However, cardiopulmonary bypass procedures with constant reinfusion of autologous blood appear to be acceptable, and several reports suggest that immediate reinfusion of salvaged autologous blood may also be acceptable to Jehovah's Witnesses.[44,45] Fortunately, considerable experience in surgical care of these patients indicates that judicious use of crystalloids frequently suffices.[46,47]

Elective Donation for Autologous Transfusion (EDAT)

General Description

Autologous blood components certainly constitute the ideal materials for elective blood transfusion. Were it not for the cost and the logistic problems entailed, all healthy people might well be urged to donate blood for themselves.

While it seems impractical to apply EDAT to the general population, the technic is indicated for several groups of people. A patient's blood can be stored in the liquid state, if needed, for an imminent transfusion or can be frozen, if long-term storage is necessary.

Short-term liquid-state storage is indicated for two types of patients:

1. Persons scheduled for elective surgery procedures that are usually associated with a significant blood loss. Included among this group are

patients with known blood group alloantibodies which may make finding compatible homologous donors difficult, and those individuals religiously opposed to homologous transfusion.

2. Persons about to undergo cardiopulmonary bypass surgery, of a type requiring the removal of blood to achieve hemodilution.

Long-term storage of blood or components in the frozen state is indicated in the following patients:

1. Persons who are alloimmunized to a very common, or "public" blood group antigen, or, whose blood contains multiple blood group isoantibodies, but who do not require an immediate transfusion.

2. Patients who are in remission from a malignant disease, and who may require concentrates of granulocytes, platelets, and/or bone marrow stem cells at some future time.

These indications for EDAT use will be discussed in more detail below. The guidelines and restrictions concerning EDAT differ in a number of respects from those which relate to the blood donor qualifications used to draw blood for homologous transfusion. Since these differences most frequently relate to short-term blood storage in the liquid state, they will be described in the section dealing with preoperative elective donation for autologous transfusion.

Preoperative EDAT (Short-Term Storage in the Liquid State)

Almost all patients who undergo elective surgery are candidates for EDAT; most underlying surgical diseases do not contraindicate the procedure. Several studies have shown strong evidence that preoperative donation for autologous transfusion is safe and practical.[48,49]

Preoperative EDAT procedures require consent by the patient's physician and an informed written consent by the patient (or, when applicable, by his parent or guardian). The consent form should also include a statement that if a unit of blood is not used for autologous transfusion, and it meets the standard criteria for donated blood, the unit can be used in homologous transfusion procedures.

Units drawn for autologous transfusion must be properly identified to ensure that the patient-donor receives his own blood. [11,50,51] In addition to conventional blood donor and recipient records, the American Association of Blood Banks recommends that a green tag be used to label the patient-donor unit at the time of collection.[51]

Each blood bank or transfusion service participating in a preoperative program for EDAT should have a written procedure manual and appropriate consent forms and labels. The procedure manual must be approved by the transfusion service's medical director and it should be consistent with the most recent edition of the American Association of Blood Banks'

Standards for Blood Banks and Transfusion Services. Deviations from the procedure manual should be undertaken only with the knowledge and approval of the transfusion service medical director and, whenever possible, the patient's physician.

The criteria for preoperative EDAT are somewhat more lenient than those established for routine blood donation.[50,51] If an EDAT blood unit does not meet all the medical criteria established for routine blood donation to protect prospective recipients, the unit must be labeled "For Autologous Use Only." These units should be separated to prevent inadvertent use in other patients; this is particularly necessary if the blood was collected from a patient with a history of hepatitis, or a positive test for HBsAg. If these units are not used by the patient-donor, they should be promptly destroyed.

Criteria for preoperative EDAT blood collection that differ from standard blood donation qualifications include:

1. There are no age restrictions; successful EDAT programs in children have been described.[52, 53]

2. There are no minimum weight requirements as long as the amount of blood collected at any one donation does not exceed 12% of the donor's body weight. When the volume of the collected blood is less than 405 ml, the volume of anticoagulant left in the blood collection container must be proportionately reduced. The volume to be removed can be calculated using the following formula:

$$VR = NV \left(1 - \frac{BD}{450*} \right)$$

* or 500, if 500-ml draw pack is used

VR = volume to be removed
NV = normal anticoagulant volume for the blood container
BD = blood to be drawn—as calculated from donor's weight × 12%

3. Uncomplicated pregnancy does not contraindicate preoperative EDAT.

4. It is possible to draw blood from patient-donors whose hematocrit is below the minimum requirement for routine blood donation. However, unless the autologous pre-donations are being collected because of extreme difficulty in finding compatible donors, phlebotomy is not performed on individuals with a hematocrit below 34%, or a hemoglobin below 11 gm/dl.

When mildly anemic patients are acting as their own donors, or whenever multiple phlebotomies are performed over a relatively short time span, supplemental iron (60 mg to 100 mg elemental iron) should be given orally three times a day. Parenteral iron offers no advantages over oral iron supplementation except in the rare patient with malabsorption.[54, 55]

While autologous units are processed and stored in the same manner as standard donor units, blood used only for autologous transfusion does not require testing for unexpected antibodies and HBsAg.[50] Compatibility testing needs remain moot. Verification of major blood group and Rh type is probably sufficient.

The frequency of preoperative collection is determined by the number of units required for the surgical procedure, and the time available for collection and storage. Whenever circumstances permit, the interval between donations, and the period from the last donation until the time of surgery should be at least 72 hours.

If the planned surgery is likely to require administration of a large number of units, the "Leap-Frog" technic first described by Ascari et al can be used.[51, 56] Using this schedule, six units are obtained, four of which (H, I, J, K) are less than nine days old. Except for the initial unit drawn, each donation is carried out using a double plasmapheresis set. When two units are being collected, one is drawn before, and one after the "reinfusion unit" is administered. As stated earlier, patient-donors entered into a Leap Frog program must take oral iron medication, three times a day.

A Leap Frog collection schedule is detailed in the following chart:

EDAT Program Day	Units(s) Drawn	Unit Infused
1	A	None
6-7	B, C	A
11-13	D, E	B
16-18	F, G	C
21-23	H, I	D
26-29	J, K	E

When larger amounts of blood are required, or when it is not feasible to collect a sufficient number of units within a four- to six-week period, one of the two units collected can be frozen. The introduction of CPD-adenine, with its 35-day shelf life, will make possible collection of larger amounts of blood for storage at 1 to 6 C.

The concern that patients entering on EDAT program will come to surgery in a significantly less optimal condition has been largely allayed by the experience with large numbers of patients over the past decade.[10] A patient subjected to preoperative phlebotomy arrives at surgery with: 1) a somewhat right-shifted oxygen dissociation curve secondary to his mild anemia; and 2) a bone marrow in a state of maximal hematopoiesis.

These conditions can both be helpful to the patient who hemorrhages acutely during major surgery. Furthermore, if the patient-donor takes iron supplements as directed, the fall in hemoglobin, which might be anticipated from an active phlebotomy program, rarely materializes.[57] Most patients whose hemoglobin is in the normal range at the start of the preoperative phlebotomy program come to surgery with hemoglobin concentrations above 10 gm/dl.[54]

In summary, preoperative elective donation for autologous transfusion is safe and effective, and in some studies has provided for most, if not all, of the blood needs of the patient-donor.[48] The advantages of the system to the individual patient are obvious, eg, preventing the use of mismatched blood, infected blood, and blood capable of inducing alloimmunization to foreign blood group or HLA antigens.

The major drawbacks of EDAT are cost and inconvenience to the patient, neither of which is insignificant. Together, these two factors probably account for the low level of enthusiasm observed in most of the major surgical centers in the United States. Nonetheless, the positive aspects of preoperative EDAT do outweigh the drawbacks. EDAT acceptance and use appear to be increasing when patients and physicians are well informed about the advantages of the procedure.

Collection of Autologous Blood Prior to Cardiopulmonary Bypass Surgery

In recent years, a number of cardiopulmonary bypass surgery teams have found it useful to hemodilute their patients to hematocrits below 30%. This is usually accomplished in the operating suite just after induction of anesthesia and before the patient is heparinized. The procedure involves the withdrawal of one to three units of blood, and the simultaneous infusion of a mixture of colloid and crystalloid solutions.[58-60] The units of blood are collected just as they would be for a standard blood donation. If the units remain within the operating suite and are properly labeled, they need not be processed. If the blood is to be reinfused immediately following the bypass, it can usually be left standing at room temperature.

When hemodilution is accomplished without preoperative phlebotomy, a large amount of dilute blood will be in the oxygenator. Several devices are available to centrifuge and pack the red cells in the oxygenator so that between two and three units can be recovered.[33, 34, 61] It is conjectural whether the return of several units of autologous blood drawn preoperatively is better for the patient than reinfusion of packed red cells recovered from the oxygenator. It seems logical that unrefrigerated "fresh whole blood" would provide a substantially larger number of platelets than packed cells recovered from the oxygenator after bypass. While this may be true, there is little evidence of reduced postoperative bleeding in the patients receiving autologous whole blood.[10]

Controversy surrounds the effectiveness of autologous transfusion in reducing the volume of homologous blood required in open-heart surgery patients. Hallowell et al[59] and Lawson et al[62] reported a significant decrease (25% to 50%) in the volume of homologous blood administered to patients undergoing prebypass phlebotomy and postoperative autotransfusion. Pliam and associates[63] and Sherman et al[64] were unable to duplicate these results. Kaplan et al[65] evaluated three methods of autotransfusion in an attempt to settle the controversy. Two of the study groups were phlebotomized prior to heparinization; one from an artery and one from a vein; and the third group was phlebotomized via a vena cava cannula after heparinization. The need for banked blood products decreased 18% in the three groups of autotransfused patients, without significant differences between them in this regard. Platelet counts rose to almost normal levels in the heparinized autotransfusion group, and blood collection was facilitated, leading to the conclusion that phlebotomy of heparinized blood from a major-vessel cannula was the method of choice. The procedure not only provided the blood use advantages of autotransfusion, but also provided a better product, from the hemostatic point of view. These observations duplicate those made by Lawson et al.[62]

Elective Donation for Autologous Transfusion (Long-Term or Frozen Storage)

Although there are considerable differences in the methodology and effectiveness of long-term storage of blood cells, it is now possible to store not only erythrocytes, but platelets, granulocytes and stem cells, for prolonged periods, in the frozen state. Uses for autologous concentrates of these components are becoming apparent, and it is now reasonable to consider autologous transfusion of frozen blood cells by cell type.

Frozen Red Blood Cells

Finding compatible blood for patients who are immunized against common or "public" blood group antigens, or who have multiple isoantibodies, creates a special problem for hospital and community transfusion services. While it is possible to screen large numbers of donor blood samples to find compatible units that can be glycerolized and stored in the frozen state, whenever possible, the collection of autologous blood should be undertaken to meet the needs of these individuals.

When an individual is identified as having blood group isoantibodies, which could make finding compatible blood a problem, he or she should be urged to establish a supply of autologous fresh blood, even though no imminent blood need is apparent. Huggins has referred to this as "open-ended" autologous blood collection.[11] For some people, this may be the only way to ensure the availability of compatible blood, should it ever be needed.

Blood from immunized individuals can be collected quickly, or at the usual two-month intervals. The blood should be stored in a facility where it can be processed for transfusion at any time. After a supply has been established, these persons should carry or wear a Med-Alert type of identification, indicating their immunohematologic status, the presence of a stored blood supply, and the telephone number needed to expedite processing and delivery of their blood to the transfusing facility. Probably, four to six units should be available for use by the patient, who should also be urged to donate additional units for other patients with the same antibodies. The availability of such units should be reported to the American Association of Blood Banks' Rare Donor File.

The usefulness of frozen autologous red blood cells for routine surgery was briefly alluded to as an alternative or supplement to the Leap Frog procedure for preoperative EDAT. This approach is used routinely by Huggins.[11] Brzica et al also discuss the application of blood freezing methodology to preoperative blood donations.[10] While some blood banks may find that this technic fits well into their routine operation, and some patients may prefer to "string-out" their donations (time permitting), in most instances, collection and storage of autologous blood for imminent surgery can best be accomplished without freezing.

Frozen Platelets

Although long-term storage of platelets is still experimental and imperfect, recent data clearly indicate that long-term frozen storage of platelets using dimethylsulfoxide (DMSO) or a glycerol-glucose mixture as the cryoprotectant is possible.[66, 67] Several recent studies indicate good viability and function of thawed frozen platelets.[68-70]

Patients with leukemia and other disorders characterized by intermittent bone marrow infiltration or depression often become resistant to random-donor platelet concentrates due to the development of alloantibodies to HLA or platelet antigens. Although compatible, or almost compatible, pheresis donors can be found, the search process can be expensive and tedious. An alternative approach—collecting and freezing autologous platelets during periods of hematologic remission—was recently described by Schiffer et al.[71] The study, which involved intensive plateletpheresis of leukemic patients in remission, demonstrated that clinically effective frozen platelet concentrates can be prepared. Among the patients studied, several were able to provide sufficient numbers of autologous platelet concentrates to supply their total platelet needs during their next relapse.

Granulocyte Concentrates

The effectiveness of granulocyte transfusions in the treatment of neutropenic patients with bacterial sepsis is now fairly well established.[72] Optimal methods for preparing and storing fresh granulocyte concentrates, however, are still a matter of conjecture.[73] Even less well understood are the conditions necessary to permit long-term frozen storage of granulocytes. Recent studies indicate that a cryoprotective mixture containing DMSO, hydroxyethyl starch (HES) and albumin may be useful.[74, 75] Zaroulis et al[74] have demonstrated good recovery of granulocytes frozen up to 18 weeks. The thawed white cells functioned well in dye exclusion and latex ingestion studies.

It appears from these studies that transfusion of granulocytes after long-term storage may soon be possible, duplicating successful reports following transfusion of previously frozen platelets. Since difficulties in finding HLA-compatible leukapheresis donors for septic leukemic patients are considerable, preparation of autologous granulocyte concentrates from patients during remission can be very beneficial.

Bone Marrow Stem Cells

Although bone marrow infusion has not been considered, heretofore, a transfusion in the usual sense, the recent realization that stem cells can be obtained in large numbers and with less trauma by leukapheresis has redirected our thinking. It is quite possible that the procedure of multiple bone marrow aspirations in the operating room will be replaced by a pheresis procedure in the transfusion service.

In 1964, Cavins et al published one of the earliest papers indicating the presence of primitive cells in the peripheral blood. The cells, now called colony-forming units (CFUc), were capable of repopulating marrow spaces and restoring marrow function.[76] The study further demonstrated that these stem cells retained viability after storage at -80 C in a serum-tissue culture mixture containing DMSO. A number of other studies have verified that viable CFUc can be maintained in frozen storage for up to 58 months,[77-80] and that they can be collected in adequate numbers from peripheral blood.[80, 81]

The possibility of repopulating the marrow with stored autologous stem cells has enormous potential value in patients with disorders characterized by intermittent bone marrow infiltration, or in patients in whom chemical marrow ablation, or total body irradiation, may have a therapeutic role. Study results are beginning to appear that point to the potential success of this process.

Applebaum et al demonstrated that cryopreserved autologous bone marrow hastened marrow recovery in lymphoma patients treated with high-dose chemotherapy.[78] Dicke et al infused leukemic patients with cryopreserved marrow after they had been treated with high-dose chemotherapy and supralethal total body irradiation. The pattern of hematopoietic recovery was similar to that observed in patients receiving syngeneic bone marrow transplants.[79]

Goldman et al[80, 82] and Whitaker and Bailey-Wood[83] recently described their experience in treating chronic granulocytic leukemia (CGL) patients with autologous buffy coat concentrates collected by leukapheresis during an early phase of the disease, and kept frozen for up to five years. Nine patients with CGL in transformation, or already in blastic crisis, were treated prior to transfusion, with high-dose chemotherapy occasionally supplemented by total body irradiation. Seven of the nine had rapid restoration of peripheral blood and bone marrow, characteristic of the chronic phase of CGL. The speed of recovery of circulating platelets and mature granulocytes indicated that marrow engraftment had occurred. The "remissions," in some patients maintained without therapy for 6 to 17 months, suggest that this form of therapy may significantly prolong the course of chronic granulocytic leukemia.

It is still uncertain whether peripheral blood buffy coats from individuals, other than those with CGL, contain CFUc equivalent to the number obtained by bone marrow aspiration. Korbling et al, however, have presented evidence suggesting that this may be the case.[81] If proven, this form of treatment may be applicable to lymphomas as well as to other kinds of leukemia.

Summary

In the past half-century, the usefulness of autologous transfusion has extended beyond the reinfusion of blood shed during traumatic, surgical or obstetrical hemorrhage. Autologous transfusion now includes elective donation by patients facing imminent surgery, or, whose immunohematologic status creates problems in providing homologous blood, as well as the postbypass autotransfusion of patients undergoing open-heart surgery. The advent of methods for cryopreserving the various cellular elements of the blood, collected by pheresis in concentrated form, has created new and exciting possibilities for the use of autologous blood components.

The major advantages of autologous transfusion deserve to be recapitulated:

1. The risk of blood-transmitted infection is nil.
2. Exposure to "foreign" blood group or HLA antigens is eliminated, and thus the risk of alloimmunization is nil.
3. Effective transfusion of previously alloimmunized patients is simplified.
4. The risk of untoward immunologic reactions (allergic, febrile, GVH) is eliminated, along with the risk of technical errors in typing and crossmatching.
5. Intraoperative salvage from massively hemorrhaging patients, and elective preoperative donation decrease the dependency upon homologous blood.
6. Some patients who would refuse homologous blood transfusion, because of religious beliefs, accept some forms of autologous transfusion.

Despite these advantages, and a dearth of important disadvantages, the use of autologous transfusions today remains sporadic. Considering the fact that the procedure represents the "ideal" form of transfusion, it would seem that more enthusiastic support by members of the blood bank and transfusion service communities is warranted.

References

1. Blundell J: Experiments on the transfusion of blood by the syringe. *Med Chir Trans* 9:56, 1818.
2. Highmore W: Practical remarks on an overlooked source of blood-supply for transfusion in post-partum hemorrhage. *Lancet* 1:89, 1874.
3. Butler HB: Auto-blood-transfusion in two cases of ruptured tubal pregnancy. *Am J Obstet Gynecol* 35:602, 1938.
4. Weil AM: A resume of one hundred consecutive cases of ectopic pregnancy. *Am J Obstet Gynecol* 35:602, 1938.
5. Duncan J: On reinfusion of blood in primary and other amputations. *Br Med J* 1:192, 1886.
6. Miller AG: Case of amputation at hip joint in which reinjection of blood was performed and rapid recovery took place. *Edinb Med J* 31:721, 1885.
7. Watson CM, Watson JR: Autotransfusion: review of American literature with report of two additional cases. *Am J Surg* 33:232, 1936.
8. Grant FC: Autotransfusion. *Ann Surg* 74:253, 1921.
9. Halsted WS: Reinfusion in carbonic-oxide poisoning. *NY State J Med* 33:625, 1883.

10. Brzica SM, Pineda AA, Taswell HF: Autologous blood transfusion. *Mayo Clin Proc* 51:723, 1976.
11. Kuban DJ: Autologous transfusion: an historical review, in *Autologous Transfusion*. Washington, DC, American Association of Blood Banks, 1976, pp 3-25.
12. Burch LE: Autotransfusion. *Surg Gynecol Obstet* 36:811, 1923.
13. Lewisohn R: A new and greatly simplified method of blood transfusion. *Med Rec* 89:141, 1915.
14. Davis LE, Cushing H: Experiences with blood replacement during or after major intracranial operations. *Surg Gynecol Obstet* 40:310, 1925.
15. Stager WR: Blood conservation by autotransfusion. *Arch Surg* 63:78, 1951.
16. Backer-Grondahl N: Auto-transfusion of blood. *Acta Chir Scand* 105:3, 1953.
17. Dyer RH: Intraoperative autotransfusion: A preliminary report and new method. *Am J Surg* 112:874, 1966.
18. Klebanoff G, Watkins D: A disposable autotransfusion unit. *Am J Surg* 116:475, 1968.
19. Brewster DC, Ambrosino JJ, Darling RC, et al: Intraoperative autotransfusion in major vascular surgery. *Am J Surg* 137:507, 1979.
20. Glover JL, Smith R, Yaw P, et al: Intraoperative autotransfusion: an underutilized technique. *Surgery* 80:474, 1976.
21. Bonfils-Roberts EA, Stutman L, Nealon TF Jr: Autologous blood in the treatment of intraoperative hemorrhage. *Ann Surg* 185:321, 1977.
22. Klebanoff G: Intraoperative autotransfusion with the Bentley ATS-100. *Surgery* 80:708, 1978.
23. Raines J, Buth J, Brewster DC: Intraoperative autotransfusion equipment, protocols, and guidelines. *J Trauma* 16:616, 1976.
24. Noon GP: Intraoperative autotransfusion. *Surgery* 84:719, 1978.
25. Davidson SJ: Emergency unit autotransfusion. *Surgery* 84:703, 1978.
26. Schaff HV, Hauer JM, Brawley RK: Autotransfusion in cardiac surgical patients after operation. *Surgery* 84:713, 1978.
27. Symbas PN: Extraoperative autotransfusion from hemothorax. *Surgery* 84:722, 1978.
28. Welch J, Weintraub H, Gutterman BJ, et al: Laboratory experience with a new autotransfusion device. *Arch Surg* 111:1374, 1976.
29. Johnston B, Kamath BSK, McLellan I: An autotransfusion apparatus. *Anaesthesia* 32:1020, 1977.
30. Mattox KL: Comparison of techniques of autotransfusion. *Surgery* 84:700, 1978.

31. Wilson JD, Taswell HF: Autotransfusion: Historical review and preliminary report of a new method. *Mayo Clin Proc* 43:26, 1968.

32. Wilson JD, Taswell HF, Utz DC: Autotransfusion: Urologic applications and the development of a modified irrigating fluid. *J Urol* 105:873, 1971.

33. Watson-Williams EJ, Kelly PB, Smeloff EA: A simple program of autologous transfusion to conserve isologous blood used for open heart surgery. *Transfusion* 15:520, 1975.

34. Moran JM, Babka R, Silberman S: Immediate centrifugation of oxygenator contents after cardiopulmonary bypass. *J Thorac Cardiovasc Surg* 76:510, 1978.

35. Orr M: Autotransfusion: the use of washed red cells as an adjunct to component therapy. *Surgery* 84:728, 1978.

36. Csencsitz TA, Flynn JC: Intraoperative blood salvage in spinal deformity surgery in children. *J Fla Med Assoc* 66:31, 1979.

37. Bennett SH, Geelhoed GW, Gralnick HR: Effects of autotransfusion on blood elements. *Am J Surg* 125:273, 1973.

38. Rakower SR: Blood surface interactions in extravascular salvageable blood pools. *Surg Gynecol Obstet* 145:555, 1977.

39. Goldfinger D: Complications of hemolytic transfusion reactions: Pathogenesis and therapy, in *New Approaches to Transfusion Reactions*. Washington, DC, American Association of Blood Banks, 1974.

40. Brener BJ, Raines JK, Chesney CM, et al: Intraoperative autotransfusion. *Surg Forum* 24:255, 1973.

41. Duncan SE, Edwards WH, Dale WA: Caution regarding autotransfusion. *Surgery* 76:1024, 1974.

42. Yaw PB, Sentany M, Link WJ, et al: Tumor cells carried through autotransfusion. Contraindication to intraoperative blood recovery? *JAMA* 231:490, 1975.

43. Watchtower Questions and Answers: Autotransfusion. *Watchtower,* Oct. 15, 1959, p 640.

44. Minuck M: Anesthesia and surgery for Jehovah's Witnesses. *Can Med Assoc J* 84:1187, 1961.

45. Sneierson H, Cunningham JR, Artuso DA: Autotransfusion for massive hemorrhage due to ruptured spleen in Jehovah's Witness. *NY State Med J* 67:1769, 1967.

46. Gollub S, Svigals R, Bailey CP, et al: Electrolyte solutions in surgical patients refusing transfusion. *JAMA* 215:2077, 1971.

47. Ott DA, Cooley DA: Cardiovascular surgery in Jehovah's Witnesses. Report of 542 operations without blood transfusion. *JAMA* 238:1256, 1977.

48. Milles G, Langston HT, Dalessandro W: *Autologous Transfusions.* Springfield, IL, Charles C. Thomas Co., 1971.
49. Newman MM, Hamstra R, Block M: Use of banked autologous blood in elective surgery. *JAMA* 218:861, 1971.
50. *Standards for Blood Banks and Transfusion Services,* ed 9. Washington, DC, American Association of Blood Banks, 1978, pp 32-34.
51. *Technical Manual,* ed 7. Washington, DC, American Association of Blood Banks, 1977, pp 270-278.
52. Cuello L, Vazquez E, Perez V: Autologous blood transfusion in cardiovascular surgery. *Transfusion* 7:309, 1967.
53. Cowell HR, Swickard JW: Autotransfusion in children's orthopaedics. *J Bone Joint Surg (Am)* 56:908, 1974.
54. Zuck TF, Bergin JJ: Adequacy of oral iron to support erythropoiesis during intensive phlebotomy for autologous transfusion (abstract), in *Proceedings of XIII International Transfusion Congress.* Washington, DC, 1972, p 53.
55. McCurdy PR: Oral and parenteral iron therapy: A comparison. *JAMA* 191:859, 1965.
56. Ascari WQ, Jolly PC, Thomas PA: Autologous blood transfusion in pulmonary surgery. *Transfusion* 8:111, 1968.
57. Finch S, Haskins D, Finch CA: Iron metabolism: Hematopoiesis following phlebotomy; iron as a limiting factor. *J Clin Invest* 29:1078, 1950.
58. Schechter DC, Sarot IA: Hydrokinetics of hemodilution cardiopulmonary bypass. *Dis Chest* 54:133, 1968.
59. Hallowell P, Bland JHL, Buckley MJ: Transfusion of fresh autologous blood in open-heart surgery: A method for reducing blood bank requirements. *J Thorac Cardiovasc Surg* 64:941, 1977.
60. Cohn LH, Fosberg AM, Anderson WP: The effects of phlebotomy, hemodilution and autologous transfusion on systemic oxygenation and whole blood utilization in open heart surgery. *Chest* 68:3, 1975.
61. Reeves WH, Milam J, Clark DK, et al: Effect of washing blood salvaged from oxygenator following extracorporeal circulation. *Am Sect Proc* 4:80, 1976.
62. Lawson NW, Ochsner JL, Mills NL, et al: The use of hemodilution and fresh autologous blood in open-heart surgery. *Anesth Analg* 53:672, 1974.
63. Pliam MB, McGoon DC, Tarhan S: Failure of transfusion of autologous whole blood to reduce banked-blood requirements in open-heart surgical patients. *J Thorac Cardiovasc Surg* 70:338, 1975.

64. Sherman MM, Dobnik DB, Dennis RC, et al: Autologous blood transfusion during cardiopulmonary bypass. *Chest* 70:5, 1976.
65. Kaplan JA, Cannarella C, Jones EL, et al: Autologous blood transfusion during cardiac surgery. *J Thorac Cardiovasc Surg* 74:4, 1977.
66. Kim BK, Tanoue K, Baldini MG: Storage of human platelets by freezing. *Vox Sang* 30:401, 1976.
67. Dayian G, Rowe AW: Cryopreservation of human platelets for transfusion. A glycerol-glucose, moderate rate cooling procedure. *Cryobiol* 13:1, 1976.
68. Schiffer CA, Aisner J, Wiernik PH: Clinical experience with transfusion of cryopreserved platelets. *Br J Haematol* 34:377, 1976.
69. Odink J, Brand A: Platelet preservation V. Survival, serotonin uptake velocity, and response to hypotonic stress of fresh and cryopreserved platelets. *Transfusion* 17:203, 1977.
70. Spector JI, Yarmala JA, Marchionni LD: Viability and function of platelets frozen at 2 to 3 C per minute with 4 or 5 percent DMSO and stored at −80 C for 8 months. *Transfusion* 17:8, 1977.
71. Schiffer CA, Aisner J, Wiernik PH: Frozen autologous platelet transfusion for patients with leukemia. *N Engl J Med* 299:7, 1978.
72. Berkman EM, Eisenstaedt RS, Caplan SN: Supportive granulocyte transfusion in the infected neutropenic patient. *Transfusion* 18:693, 1978.
73. Glasser L: Functional considerations of granulocyte concentrates used for clinical transfusions. *Transfusion* 19:1, 1979.
74. Zaroulis CG, Leiderman IZ, Lee SC: Freeze-preservation of human granulocytes for transfusion therapy, abstracted. *Clin Res* 27:310A, 1979.
75. French JE, Jemionek JF, Contreras TJ: Cryopreservation of dog polymorphonuclear leukocytes (PMNL) for transfusion, abstracted. *Exp Hematol* 6 (Suppl. 3):107, 1978.
76. Cavins JA, Scheer SC, Thomas ED, et al: The recovery of lethally irradiated dogs given infusions of autologous leukocytes preserved at −80 C. *Blood* 23:38, 1964.
77. Ragab AH, Gilkerson E, Myers M: Factors in the preservation of bone marrow cells from children with acute leukemia. *Cryobiol* 14:125, 1977.
78. Applebaum FR, Herzig GP, Ziegler JL, et al: Successful engraftment of cryopreserved autologous bone marrow in patients with malignant lymphoma. *Blood* 52:85, 1978.
79. Dicke KA, Spitzer G, Peters L, et al: Autologous bone-marrow transplantation in relapsed adult leukemia. *Lancet* 1:514, 1979.
80. Goldman JM, Catovsky D, Hows J, et al: Cryopreserved peripheral

blood cells functioning as autografts in patients with chronic granulocytic leukaemia in transformation. *Brit Med J* 1:1310, 1979.

81. Korbling M, Fliedner TM, Pflieger H, et al: Yield and efficiency of
collecting and cryopreserving human hemopoiteic blood stem-cells
(HBSC) by means of continuous flow centrifugation (CFC), abstracted. *Exp Hematol* 6 (Suppl. 3):95, 1968.

82. Goldman JM, Catovsky D, Galton DAG: Reversal of blast-cell
crisis in C.G.L. by transfusion of stored autologous buffy-coat cells.
Lancet 1:437, 1978.

83. Whitaker JH, Bailey-Wood R: Autologous buffy-coat cells for
chronic granulocytic leukaemia in blast-cell crisis. *Lancet* 2:1380,
1979.

Chapter 8

EXTRACORPOREAL CIRCULATION

R. Thomas Solis, MD

Introduction

IN RECENT YEARS, new technology has been developed, by which blood can be temporarily removed from the circulation—in order to alter a particular component—and then transfused for recirculation. This chapter discusses these new technics in extracorporeal circulation. In a broad sense, autologous transfusion and pheresis fall within this technological category, but because of their individual importance and usefulness, these procedures are discussed separately in Chapters 7 and 15.

Hemodialysis

Patients with advanced renal disease are often chronically anemic.[1] This anemia, which may be due to plasma volume expansion or chronically depressed erythropoiesis, may not benefit from transfusion. The few patients who do require periodic transfusions may experience enhancement of future graft survival if exposed to blood from random donors. The use of leukocyte-poor or frozen red cells is no longer considered necessary or desirable for potential transplant candidates. (This subject is discussed in further detail in Chapter 4.)

Today, artificial kidneys require no priming with donor blood and the small volume of blood remaining in the circuit can be returned to the patient after dialysis. Since the blood within the extracorporeal circuit must be anticoagulated, either systemic or "regional heparinization" of the circuit must be accomplished.[2] Hepatitis is a serious problem in hemodialysis units and rigid precautions should be taken to protect the recipients and the unit personnel. Some dialysis units have reduced the incidence of hepatitis by isolating patients who are already afflicted or are known carriers of this disease.

Heart Lung Bypass With Pump-Oxygenator[3]

Due to the large volume of blood needed in open-heart surgery, the increasing use of coronary artery bypass procedures for treatment of ischemic heart disease has placed an increasing burden on the nation's blood resources.[4] The problem is compounded by the often severe restrictions some surgeons place on the type and age of blood and blood products required during and immediately after cardiopulmonary bypass. However, since many centers have greatly reduced their average blood utilization,[5-9] one can anticipate widespread acceptance of technics that decrease the amount of blood used during open-heart surgery.

The fluid used to prime the extracorporeal circuit may be either donor blood or nonblood solutions. A major reduction in blood utilization has resulted from the increased use of hemodilution technics, which allow priming of the pump oxygenator with balanced salt solutions. The maximum amount of salt solutions that can be mixed with the blood of the patient is that which does not lower the hematocrit below 20%. Albumin or other colloid preparations may be added to preserve the plasma colloid osmotic pressure. Hemodilution, which reduces blood viscosity and may result in less red cell aggregation and better tissue perfusion, has been safely tolerated by a large number of adults undergoing both rheumatic valvular and coronary artery bypass surgery without increased mortality or morbidity.[5-9] Reducing the number of transfused units by eliminating blood from the "prime" reduces many risks to the patient (eg, red cell antibody formation, hepatitis, and the postperfusion syndrome), and simplifies the problems of supplying blood for the procedure. Because of these advantages, nonblood priming solutions should be used with most adults.

If a blood prime must be used, citrated CPD blood is employed after addition of heparin followed by recalcification. The amount of calcium used is usually 1 ml of 10% calcium gluconate per 100 ml of ACD blood and 0.8 ml per 100 ml of CPD blood. Since the citrate anticoagulants provide an extra acid load, sodium bicarbonate is frequently added. Use of citrated blood (rather than heparinized blood) for priming greatly simplifies supply problems, speeds preparations in an emergency, and prevents loss of blood, if surgery is postponed at the last minute.

Blood lost from the circulation during bypass can be replaced as citrated blood with recalcification. If massive quantities of blood are used, then blood stored less than five days should be used, as described in Chapter 6. However, many centers routinely use blood regardless of storage age without untoward effects. Frozen red cells may also be used safely during open-heart surgery,[9] and are particularly useful when the recipient has a rare blood type. One technic which has greatly reduced blood utilization is autologous transfusion. (Details of this procedure are discussed in Chapter 7.) By using such technics, some institutions have been able to reduce their average blood utilization to two to five units per case.[4] Any center that exceeds this number should carefully review its blood utilization policies.

Complications

Since patients undergoing cardiopulmonary bypass must be systematically heparinized, oozing of blood from cut surfaces is to be expected. The initial heparin dose should be at least 300 units/kg, with an additional 100 units/kg/hr in long procedures. There is no evidence that these heparin doses cause increased bleeding, but many feel that inadequate heparinization leads to consumption of fibrinogen and other hemostasis factors and, thus, increases blood loss.

It is generally accepted that postoperative complications are directly related to the time of cardiopulmonary bypass. A moderate thrombocytopenia may occur as a result of hemodilution and trapping of platelets in the microcirculation. When massive amounts of blood are given, thrombocytopenia may become severe enough to require administration of platelet concentrates to control postoperative bleeding. It must be emphasized that most patients will have platelet counts well below normal for several days after surgery, but they will not bleed.

Hepatitis is an unavoidable complication of blood transfusion. The frequency of hepatitis following heart surgery is proportional to the number of donors involved and the carrier rate in the donor population. The use of frozen red cells may be indicated to reduce the incidence of some transfusion hazards, including hepatitis, hyperkalemia, and febrile reactions.

Following multiple transfusions, alloantibodies to red cells, platelets, white cells, and plasma proteins may occur, creating a problem for the patient who requires further transfusions.

References

1. Erslev AJ: Anemia of chronic renal failure. *Arch Intern Med* 126:774, 1970.
2. Gordon LA, Simon ER, Rukes JM, et al: Studies in regional heparinization. II. Artificial kidney hemodialysis without systemic heparinization. Preliminary report of a method using simultaneous infusion of heparin and protamine. *N Engl J Med* 255:1063, 1956.
3. National Academy of Sciences-National Research Council: Summary of the proceedings of a conference on the use of blood and blood substitutes for extracorporeal circulation. *Transfusion* 6:355, 1966.
4. Roche JK, Stengle JM: Open-heart surgery and the demand for blood. *JAMA* 225:1516, 1973.
5. Cooley DA, Beall AC Jr., Grondin P: Open-heart operations with disposable oxygenators, 5 percent dextrose prime, and normothermia. *Surgery* 52:713, 1962.

6. Zubiate P, Kay JH, Mendex AM, et al: Coronary artery surgery: A new technique with use of little blood, if any. *J Thorac Cardiovasc Surg* 68:263, 1974.
7. Sandiford FM, Chiariello L, Hallman GL, et al: Aortocoronary bypass in Jehovah's Witnesses. *J Thorac Cardiovasc Surg* 68:1, 1974.
8. Verska JJ, Ludington LG, Brewer LA: A comparative study of cardiopulmonary bypass with nonblood and blood prime. *Ann Thorac Surg* 18:72, 1974.
9. Cohn LH, Fosberg AM, Anderson WP, et al: The effects of phlebotomy, hemodilution and autologous transfusion on systemic oxygenation and whole blood utilization in open-heart surgery. *Chest* 68:3, 1975.

Chapter 9

PLATELET TRANSFUSIONS

John T. Crosson, MD

Introduction

TRANSFUSION OF PLATELETS is meant to temporarily improve hemostasis defects in patients lacking an adequate number of hemostatically effective platelets. At the present time, such transfusions can be accomplished effectively by using platelet concentrates. A platelet concentrate may be prepared from a single unit of blood and usually contains more than 0.6×10^{11} platelets; up to 7×10^{11} platelets can be harvested from a single donor using current automated plateletpheresis technics.

Storage

Platelets must be stored in such a manner that they survive and function optimally when transfused. Since stored platelets undergo morphologic changes leading to aggregation and decreased survival in vivo, when the pH drops below 6.0, the storage conditions must assure a pH above this critical level. Therefore, platelets from a single unit that are stored at 22 C should be resuspended in 50 ml of plasma.[1,2]

Although some investigators have previously reported improved hemostasis with storage temperatures of 4 C,[3,5] this procedure is now generally discredited and is no longer in use.[4] If, however, platelets are stored at 4 C for the possible improved hemostatic effect, they should not be stored for more than 24 hours and can be resuspended in 20 ml of plasma. The survival of platelets stored at 22 C up to 72 hours is satisfactory, provided that they are agitated gently.[6]

Platelets collected by automated plateletpheresis are resuspended in 40 ml to 60 ml plasma for each 1×10^{11} platelets. Since collection does not take place in a closed system, the platelets must be transfused within 24 hours. If necessary, such platelets can be concentrated further just prior to transfusion.

Indications for Transfusion

The decision to initiate a platelet transfusion must be based on an assessment of the clinical state of the patient (ie, signs of bleeding, petechiae, ecchymosis); laboratory data (ie, platelet counts, bone marrow studies, platelet function tests); and anticipated future needs of the patient. For example, thrombocytopenic patients (less than 20,000/cmm) with impaired platelet production and clinical signs of bleeding may benefit from platelet transfusions. Spontaneous bleeding in such patients is rare when platelet counts are in excess of 20,000/cmm.[7] However, many patients may have platelet counts less than 20,000/cmm for long periods of time without clinical bleeding. These patients generally do not need exogenous platelets. Similarly, thrombocytopenic patients with single bleeding sites that can be controlled locally may not need platelet transfusions.

Platelet-related bleeding of any kind is rare with platelet counts greater than 75,000 to 100,00/cmm.[8] A thrombocytopenic patient suffering traumatic injuries or requiring major surgery ideally should receive a platelet transfusion calculated to elevate his platelet count to such a level. Because of rapid consumption at bleeding sites, peripheral platelet counts may not show the anticipated rise. In many instances, adequate hemostasis is achieved in these situations if the platelet count is maintained at 50,000/cmm.

Several studies have indicated that prophylactic use of platelet transfusions in patients lacking clinical signs of bleeding, but with platelet counts less than 10,000 to 20,000/cmm, prevents the development of hemorrhage and reduces morbidity and mortality. It must be remembered, however, that patients may tolerate platelet counts as low as 5,000/cmm without developing any bleeding complications. Therefore, in deciding whether to administer prophylactic platelet transfusions, one must weigh the risks of possible disease transmission or sensitization to platelet or HLA antigens against the presumed risk of bleeding.

Platelet transfusions should not be administered to patients with rapid destruction of platelets (as in idopathic thrombocytopenic purpura, disseminated lupus erythematosus, vasculitis or drug-induced thrombocytopenia), unless there is severe life-threatening hemorrhage, since transfused platelets are destroyed as rapidly as the patient's own platelets and, therefore, have a transient effect, at most. Such patients frequently tolerate the thrombocytopenic state well; they will respond to steroids and their platelet counts will improve. As the use of platelets from single donors becomes more widespread, concepts regarding use of platelets in these "consumptive" diseases may change.

Certain patients with qualitative platelet defects, due either to inherited disorders or certain drugs, may require platelet transfusions for clinical bleeding even if the platelet count is normal. In the absence of a simple and reliable laboratory test for platelet function, the template modification of the Ivy bleeding time probably provides the best means of assessing the need for transfusion in these patients.[8]

Compatibility Testing and Sensitization

Platelet concentrates need not be crossmatched prior to administration. Platelets carry the ABO antigens; in order to obtain the best recovery of transfused platelets, some authorities recommend that platelets should be ABO-compatible, while others feel this is not necessary. ABO-incompatible platelets are clearly hemostatically of benefit to the recipient. However, the compatibility of the donor plasma with the recipient red cells must be considered. Since 50 ml of plasma remains in each platelet concentrate, enough anti-A or anti-B may be passively administered to ABO-incompatible individuals to produce a positive direct Coombs test and hemolytic anemia. Therefore, infants, in particular, should receive only ABO-specific platelets because of their small blood volume and the relatively large amount of plasma which might be infused when platelets are given. Since platelets do not carry the Rh antigens, Rh sensitization can only arise from contaminating red cells, which are usually present in the platelet concentrates. The risk of such sensitization is low[11] and, when clinically indicated, can usually be prevented with the use of Rh-immune globulin.

Patients receiving multiple platelet transfusions from random donors frequently become sensitized to platelet antigens, resulting in a markedly shortened survival rate of subsequently transfused platelets. The frequency of this refractory state increases in proportion to the number of platelet transfusions a patient receives. For this reason, only the number of platelets needed to produce the desired clinical result should be given. In most situations, four to six donor units are satisfactory. Platelets from related HLA-identical donors transfused into patients completely refractory to random donors have near normal survival,[12] demonstrating the relationship of the HLA system to platelet survival. Platelets from unrelated HLA-identical or closely-matched donors produce similar results.[14] There are some refractory patients who do not respond to HLA-matched platelets, indicating that antigen systems, perhaps specific to platelets, outside the HLA system can lead to sensitization and the refractory state.

Generally, patients requiring long-term platelet support periodically receive platelet concentrates from random donors. An alternative approach is to use platelets obtained from a limited number of random donors by automated plateletpheresis. If a patient becomes sensitized, as demonstrated by markedly decreased survival of transfused platelets, then HLA-matched unrelated or related donors will have to be used. Approximately four to eight units of platelets can be obtained from one donor during automated plateletpheresis. Therefore, one or two HLA-matched donors can usually provide adequate platelets for a sensitized recipient. Platelets obtained by plateletpheresis technics usually include enough red cells to make red cell compatibility important. Furthermore, platelets collected by plateletpheresis must be used within 24 hours.

Administration

Platelets from donors of the same ABO group may either be pooled into a single transfer bag or syringe for administration or they may be administered as individual units. Several platelet administration sets are available for use. All have a standard 170μ filter, which should always be used when giving platelets. Filters designed to remove particles less than 170μ (microaggregate filters) cannot be used (with the possible exception of the Pall filter), since they remove a moderate number of platelets as well. Standard blood administration sets with 170μ filters are acceptable. As long as platelets are carefully resuspended after centrifugation and gently agitated during storage, very few platelets will be removed by a filter this size. It is advisable to use a 19-gauge needle or larger for administration. Platelets should be administered rapidly, within an average of five minutes per platelet concentrate. Occasionally, a patient's clinical response will be better if the platelets are "dripped" in slowly rather than administered rapidly. Isotonic saline should be used to flush the container and filter to insure maximum infusion of the platelets.

Monitoring platelet transfusions is difficult and no one single method is satisfactory. Generally, one platelet concentrate will produce an increment of about 7,000 platelets per cmm one hour after transfusions in a 70-kg adult (about 100/cmm/kg). However, many factors (eg, splenomegaly, previous sensitization, fever, sepsis and active bleeding), influence recovery and survival of transfused platelets. Thus, a failure to achieve the expected increment does not necessarily indicate ineffectiveness of the transfusion.

The best laboratory method to assess effectiveness of platelet transfusions is to follow improvement of the template modification of the Ivy bleeding time. This, however, is not always practical. Although not quantitative, evaluation of the general clinical response (including cessation of active bleeding and resolution of ecchymosis) provides an important and necessary means of monitoring platelet transfusions. Since drugs present in the circulation of patients can alter the function of transfused platelets, thrombocytopenic patients should not receive drugs known to adversely affect platelet function, eg, aspirin and some antihistamines.

Thus, in deciding how many platelets to administer to a given patient, one must take into consideration the size of the patient, the desired increment in the platelet count, the presence of factors known to decrease survival and the general clinical response of the patient. Excessive use of multidonor platelets is to be avoided; nonimmunized adult patients will frequently stop bleeding with four units. Another factor to consider when deciding dosage is that, although storage times up to 72 hours are generally accepted, there is evidence that platelets stored for shorter periods yield better recoveries and are hemostatically more effective.[1,2]

Consumption of platelets in the extracorporeal circulation apparatus in patients who are having open-heart surgery will often occur. If such consumption is of a magnitude to require platelet administration (less than 50,000/cmm), the platelets should only be given after the patient has been taken off the extracorporeal circulation in order to avoid unnecessary destruction of transfused platelets. There is no benefit to using prophylactic platelets under these circumstances.[12]

Complications

When deciding whether or not a patient needs a platelet transfusion, it must be remembered that serious and diverse complications can develop with the use of platelet concentrates. It is important, therefore, to carefully document the indications for platelet transfusions in a given patient and to transfuse *only* when definitely required for the benefit of the patient.

Complications arising from platelet transfusion are similar to those arising from the transfusion of other blood components (see Chapter 14); therefore, only those problems unique to platelet transfusions will be discussed here. The hepatitis risk from one unit of platelet concentrate is likely to be the same as the risk from a unit of whole blood. When it is realized that thrombocytopenic patients often receive multiple units of platelet concentrates, the increased risk of hepatitis development in these patients can be appreciated.

Allergic reactions, while usually not serious, can occur with platelet concentrates. Reactions to plasma proteins, in particular to IgA with the propensity to produce anaphylaxis, occur with platelet concentrates. Although a single unit contains only 50 ml of plasma, many patients receive up to eight units at a time and, thus, receive as much plasma as contained in a unit of whole blood.

All platelet concentrates contain some leukocytes and, therefore, are capable of producing leukocyte-initiated reactions, eg, febrile reactions, similar to those produced with whole blood. Also, severely immuno-suppressed patients can theoretically suffer graft-versus-host reactions. This potentially lethal problem can be avoided by irradiation of plate-let concentrates with 1500 to 3000 rad. Since small quantities of red cells, as well as leukocytes, are present in platelet concentrates, sensitization to red cell antigens can occur.

As stated previously, patients can become refractory to platelet transfusions because of sensitization to platelet antigens, some of which are identical to or closely linked to the HLA antigens. Furthermore, platelet transfusions in patients who are sensitized to specific platelet antigens can produce definite clinical symptoms, including chills, fever and headache. Febrile reactions to platelets have been reported to occur in 2% to 5% of all patients.

Bacteremia following transfusion of platelets stored at room temperature has been reported.[16] Though this is rare, the possibility should be considered in patients who develop a fever following platelet transfusion.

References

1. Murphy S, Sayer S, Gardner F: Storage of platelet concentrates at 22 C. *Blood* 35:549, 1970.
2. Murphy S, Gardner F: Platelet preservation. *N Engl J Med* 280:1094, 1969.
3. Becker G, Tucelli M, Kunicki T, et al: Studies of platelet concentrates stored at 22 C and 4 C. *Transfusion* 13:61, 1973.
4. Slichter S, Harker L: Preparation and storage of platelet concentrates. *Transfusion* 16:8, 1976.
5. Valeri C: Circulation and hemostatic effectiveness of platelets stored at 4 C or 22 C. *Transfusion* 16:20, 1976.
6. Proceedings—Platelet Concentrate Workshop, Bethesda, MD, Jan. 5, 1978.
7. Gyados L, Freireich E, Mantel N: The quantitative relation between platelet count and hemorrhage in patients with acute leukemia. *N Engl J Med* 266:905, 1962.
8. Harker L, Slichter S: The bleeding time as a screening test for evaluation of platelet function. *N Engl J Med* 287:155, 1972.
9. Highby DJ, Cohen E, Holland JF, et al: The prophylactic treatment of thrombocytopenic leukemia patients with platelets. *Transfusion* 14:440, 1974.
10. Murphy S, Koch PA, Evans AE: Randomized trial of prophylactic vs. therapeutic platelet transfusion in childhood acute leukemia. *Clin Res* 24:379a, 1976.
11. Goldfinger D, McGinniss M: Rh incompatible platelet trans-

fusions—Risks and consequences of sensitizing immunosuppressed patients. *N Engl J Med* 284:942, 1971.

12. Yankee R, Grumet F, Rogentine G: Platelet transfusion therapy—Selection of compatible platelet donors for refractory patients by lymphocyte HL-A typing. *N Engl J Med* 281:1208, 1969.

13. Harding SA, Shakoor MA, Grindon AJ: Platelet support for cardio-pulmonary bypass surgery. *J Thorac Cardiovasc Surg* 70:350, 1975.

14. Lohrmann H, Bull M, Decter J, et al: Platelet transfusions from HL-A compatible unrelated donors to alloimmunized patients. *Ann Intern Med* 80:9, 1974.

15. Aster R, Becker G, Filip D: Studies to improve methods of short term platelet preservation. *Transfusion* 16:4, 1976.

16. Bucholz D, et al: Bacterial proliferation in platelet products stored at room temperature. *N Engl J Med* 285:429, 1971.

17. Aisner J: Platelet transfusion therapy. *Med Clin North Am* 61:1133, 1977.

Chapter 10

GRANULOCYTE TRANSFUSION
AND BONE MARROW TRANSPLANTATION

John T. Crosson, MD

Granulocyte Transfusions

WHILE THE USE of platelet concentrates in the treatment of hemorrhagic complications due to thrombocytopenia is standard practice, the use of granulocyte transfusions in leukopenic states has just recently achieved widespread use. Most studies have indicated that granulocyte transfusion during an infectious episode in a leukopenic patient is likely to help the patient recover from the infection.[1-9] In one study, however, the efficacy of granulocyte transfusion was questioned, since the control group did as well as the treated group.[10]

Higby recently analyzed a group of controlled granulocyte transfusion studies reported in the literature.[11] He observed that survivors in the control group, but not in the transfused group, generally showed signs of early bone marrow recovery (82%). Compared to nontransfused patients with delay in recovering bone marrow function, patients receiving granulocyte transfusions who did not have rapid bone marrow recovery clearly had improved survival rates. Since there is no reliable means of identifying those patients who will recover bone marrow function, it seems reasonable to provide granulocyte transfusions for severely infected neutropenic patients, if possible.

Preparations of granulocytes from normal donors by continuous or intermittent centrifugation leukapheresis generally contain about $5-8 \times 10^9$ granulocytes per donation. The use of a red cell sedimenting agent such as hydroxyethyl starch (HES)[12] will increase the yield to $10-12 \times 10^9$. If steroids are used with HES, the yield will be as high as $2-3 \times 10^{10}$. Filtration leukapheresis, on the other hand, generally yields concentrates with from 2 to 5×10^{10} granulocytes. Both technics yield products satisfactory for clinical use and there is no definite data indicating the superiority of one over the other. Although the peripheral blood white cell increments seen in patients transfused with leukocytes obtained by filtration leukapheresis are less than with other methods, this probably is of no clinical importance. Since the granulocytes' functional activity is at the site of infection rather than in the circulation, increments in peripheral blood white counts are not important in evaluating efficacy of the transfusion. There is some in vitro evidence, however, that the function of filtered cells in phagocytic and bactericidal tests may be somewhat decreased.[3,13,14]

Preparations from patients with chronic myelogenous leukemia have also been used for granulocyte transfusions. Buffy coat preparations collected from single donations from a normal donor do not contain enough granulocytes to be effective.

The decision whether or not to give granulocyte transfusions should be carefully thought out since the leukapheresis procedure is time-consuming for the donor and potentially dangerous to him, and effective therapy for a neutropenic patient may require daily leukocyte transfusions for at least five days or longer.[1] While granulocyte transfusions generally should be reserved as short-term support for patients with transient leukopenia, patients with aplastic anemia who develop an acute infection might benefit from a course of leukocyte transfusions. Clinical criteria for white cell transfusion may vary from hospital to hospital, but they should be well established and agreed on by all involved individuals before a leukocyte transfusion program is initiated. Such criteria might include a granulocyte count less than 500/cmm, fever over 38.5 C, clinical and laboratory evidence of infection, and failure to respond to antibiotics in 48 hours. Furthermore, because of potential dangers to the donor, a strict donor screening protocol should be established and followed.

Criteria for selection of donors include the following: (1) age limits of 18 to 66; (2) no medical contraindication to anticoagulation or routine blood donation (especially the absence of hypertension); and (3) a signed consent form.

Minor alterations in donor blood counts, including a fall in hemoglobin levels by about 1 gm% and an initial fall in granulocyte counts followed by a rise at the end of the procedure are frequently seen.[3,15] Filtration leukapheresis may result in a drop in donor platelets to 50% of the initial level by the end of the procedure.

Because of the time commitment of the donor, many centers depend on family members or friends for leukocyte concentrates. Donors should be ABO-compatible with the patient. HLA compatibility is of importance only with respect to allosensitization. If the patient is a potential bone marrow transplant recipient, he should not receive leukocytes or other blood components from family members because of the risk of sensitization to minor histocompatibility antigens shared by the potential donor. It is desirable to check the patient's serum for the presence of agglutinating antibodies directed against the donor white cells. If a recipient develops leukoagglutinins directed against the donor white cells, subsequent granulocyte transfusions should probably be obtained from a different donor. Since red cells are always present in a leukocyte concentrate from continuous flow leukapheresis, the standard red cell crossmatch should also be performed.

Leukocyte concentrates are indicated daily for at least four or five days, or until a satisfactory clinical response is observed. Longer periods of transfusion may be beneficial for patients who do not respond immediately.[11] Therapy with granulocyte concentrates should be started by at least one to two days after onset of infection and the leukocyte dose should be around 1.5×10^{10} for preparations obtained by centrifugation methods. Such concentrates should be administered through a standard 170μ filter slowly over two to four hours, since more rapid infusion may cause severe pulmonary reactions. No reliable laboratory methods exist to monitor these transfusions. Though 10% of administered cells are frequently recovered in the peripheral blood one hour after transfusion, failure to achieve this expected increment in white cell count does not indicate that the transfusion has been ineffective. The best way to monitor the transfusion is by careful documentation of the clinical course, looking for lysis of fever and improvement of the infection. Migration of granulocytes into skin chambers seems to be a worthwhile, but difficult, way to monitor the efficacy in vivo of granulocyte transfusions.

It is not known whether or not prophylactic granulocytes are of any value in neutropenic patients without infections. A prospective study is underway to evaluate this.

Besides the usual complications associated with administration of blood products, certain complications are particularly likely to be seen with leukocyte transfusion. Among the most frequently occurring complications are febrile reactions, seen in one-half to two-thirds of patients undergoing leukocyte transfusion.[5] Patients with severe chills and fever during transfusion may be given Demerol, 25 to 75 mg IV. This stops the chills rapidly, but does not alter the fever. Respiratory insufficiency has been seen on rare occasions, but is prevented by slow infusion.

Graft-versus-host reactions are a hazard of granulocyte transfusions because the recipients are almost always pancytopenic secondary to cytotoxic therapy, which is also immunosuppressive. Graft-versus-host disease is less likely to occur when granulocytes are prepared by filtration leukapheresis (as compared with the other methods) because filtration leukapheresis yields primarily granulocytes and less than 5% lymphocytes. Since the totally immunosuppressed patient may be more likely to develop this severe complication, granulocytes administered to such individuals can be irradiated with 1500 to 3000 rads, which presumably inhibits the function of lymphocytes without altering the function of the granulocytes. Since red cells are present in leukocyte concentrates, sensitization to red cell antigens is theoretically possible.

Bone Marrow Transplantation

Bone marrow transplantation is a relatively new, highly experimental therapeutic approach which is presently limited to a few major medical centers. Patients with some forms of immunodeficiency diseases can frequently be dramatically helped with bone marrow transplantation. Chronic aplastic anemia may be cured with transplantation. Four-year survival rates of aplastic anemia patients receiving bone marrow transplants in Seattle are about 45%.[17,20] Without transplantation, such patients all expire within a year. Paroxysmal nocturnal hemoglobinuria is occasionally an indication for bone marrow transplantation. Though patients with acute hematologic malignancies present unique problems regarding complete eradication of the malignant cells by irradiation, recent reports of relatively long-term survivors among acute leukemia patients who have had successful bone marrow transplants following cyclophosphamide treatment and total irradiation are very encouraging.[18,19] In a few patients, however, the leukemia has been shown to be present in the transplanted cells several months after transplantation.

Most bone marrow transplants have been done using HLA-identical, ABO-compatible and mixed lymphocyte culture unreactive siblings. Several ABO-incompatible transplants have been done with success, however, indicating that ABO matching, in contrast to other organ allografts, is not required for bone marrow transplantation. The need for rigid histocompatibility in the HLA system obviously excludes many potential recipients who might otherwise be good candidates.

Potential bone marrow recipients should not receive red blood cells or other blood components from the potential donor or from other family members, even if HLA identical, because of the risk of sensitization to minor histocompatibility antigens. Transfusions from random donors have also been shown to lead to sensitization and, therefore, transfusions should be kept to a minimum. Such sensitization has been shown to increase the risk of rejection of engrafted marrow, both experimentally and in humans.[20]

Because of the large volumes of bone marrow required (250 cc to 900 cc) the donor needs to be anesthetized during the aspiration from multiple sites. After appropriate processing, the marrow is then injected intravenously into the recipient.

Complications are seen frequently in patients receiving bone marrow transplantation. While the incidence of graft rejection has declined through improved compatibility testing and immunosuppressive therapy, it still occurs frequently enough to be considered a major problem (30% in patients with aplastic anemia).[17] Graft-versus-host (GVH) disease, however, is an extremely common problem (about 70% of bone marrow recipients),[18] and adequate control technics for this serious problem are still lacking. Such reactions have proven fatal in 10% to 20% of human bone marrow recipients. There is some evidence that X and Y chromosomes may contribute to GVH and, therefore, sex matching may be important.[20]

In order to eliminate donor lymphocytes capable of producing GVH disease, it is important to irradiate (1,500 to 3,000 rads) all blood products which are to be infused into bone marrow recipients during their immuno-incompetent phase. Recurrent leukemia during the first two years posttransplantation is a common cause of death. It has been estimated that about two-thirds of patients with leukemia who receive a bone marrow transplant will develop recurrent leukemia within two years. It may be possible to reduce the incidence of recurrent leukemia by transplanting during remission or by more intensive anti-leukemic therapy.[19] There are a number of opportunistic infections that can present major problems for these patients. One of the most serious is cytomegalovirus. This has been implicated in a high proportion of patients with interstitial pneumonitis and can be fatal. Other agents which produce serious infections include Pneumocystis carinii and herpes simplex.

Because of the complexity of compatibility testing and the risks involved in bone marrow transplantation, these procedures can only be performed in centers with experienced staff. It is essential for potential recipients to be identified early so that proper preparative treatment can be given and testing arrangements can be made early in the patient's course.

References

1. Graw, R, Herzig G, Perry S, et al: Normal granulocyte transfusion therapy. Treatment of septicemia due to gram negative bacteria. *N Engl J Med* 287:367, 1972.
2. McCredie K, Freireich E, Hester J, et al: Leukocyte transfusion therapy for patients with host-defense failure. *Transplant Proc* 5:1285, 1973.
3. Highby D, Yates J, Henerson E, et al: Filtration leukaphesesis for granulocyte transfusion therapy. *N Engl J Med* 292:761, 1975.
4. Lowenthal R, Goldman J, Buskord N, et al: Granulocyte transfusions in treatment of patients with acute leukemia and aplastic anemia. *Lancet* 1:353, 1975.

5. Schifter C, Buchholz D, Aisner J, et al: Clinical experience with transfusion of granulocytes obtained by continuous flow filtration leukapheresis. *Am J Med* 58:373, 1975.

6. Herzig RH, Herzig GP, Graw RG, et al: Successful granulocyte transfusion therapy for gram negative septicemia. A prospectively randomized controlled study. *N Engl J Med* 296:701, 1977.

7. Alavi JB, Root RK, Djerassi I, et al: A randomized clinical trial of granulocyte transfusions for infection in acute leukemia. *N Engl J Med* 296:706, 1977.

8. Vogler WR, Winton EF: A controlled study of the efficacy of granulocyte transfusions in patients with neutropenia. *Am J Med* 63:548, 1977.

9. Clift RA, Sanders JE, Thomas ED, et al: Granulocyte transfusions for the prevention of infection in patients receiving bone marrow transplants. *N Engl J Med* 298:1052, 1978.

10. Fortuny I, Bloomfield C, Hadlock D, et al: Granulocyte transfusion: A controlled study in patients with acute nonlymphocytic leukemia. *Transfusion* 15:548, 1975.

11. Higby D: Controlled prospective studies of granulocyte transfusion therapy. Presented at Leukocyte Symposium, London, England, 1976.

12. Mishler J, Hadlock D, Fortuny I, et al: Increased efficiency of leukocyte collection by the addition of hydroxyethyl starch to the continuous-flow centrifuge. *Blood* 44:571, 1974.

13. Herzig G, Root R, Graw R: Granulocyte collection by continuous-flow filtration leukapheresis. *Blood* 39:554, 1972.

14. McCullough J et al: In vitro function and post-transfusion survival of granulocytes collected by continuous-flow centrifugation and by filtration leukapheresis. *Blood* 48:315, 1976.

15. Russell J, Powles, B: *Clin Hematol* 5:81, 1976.

16. Mass M, Dean P, Weston W, et al: Leukocyte migration in vivo: A new method of study. *J Lab Clin Med* 86:1040, 1975.

17. Storb R: Aplastic anemia treated by allogeneic marrow transplantation, in *Human Bone Marrow Transplantation*. Washington, D. C., American Association of Blood Banks, p 35, 1976.

18. Thomas ED et al: Bone marrow transplantation. *N Engl J Med* 292:832, 895, 1975.

19. Sanders JE, Thomas ED: Bone marrow transplantation for acute leukemia. *Clin Haematol* 7:295, 1978.

20. Storb R, Thomas ED: Marrow transplantation for treatment of aplastic anemia. *Clin Haematol* 7:597, 1978.

Chapter 11

TRANSFUSION OF PLASMA AND PLASMA DERIVATIVES, INCLUDING ALBUMIN

R. Thomas Solis, MD, David Smith, MD
Lewellys F. Barker, MD

Single Donor Plasma Products

SINGLE DONOR PLASMA can be obtained by centrifugation or sedimentation of a unit of whole blood and removal of the supernatant plasma, or by phasmapheresis. The product has a volume of approximately 200 ml to 250 ml. The labile coagulation Factors V and VIII will deteriorate during storage at 4 C. Single donor plasma differs, therefore, from single donor fresh frozen plasma primarily in its lower concentration of these two factors. According to federal regulations, single donor plasma can be stored in the liquid state for no more than 26 days from the date of collection in a plastic bag and can be stored frozen for no more than five years.

If the plasma from a unit of whole blood is separated from the red blood cells within six hours of collection and frozen rapidly, the plasma product is then called single donor fresh frozen plasma. Freezing arrests the deterioration of the labile coagulation factors. If the single donor fresh frozen plasma is transfused within two hours of thawing, it will be as therapeutically effective as single donor freshly drawn plasma in correcting coagulation defects due to a deficiency of the labile clotting factors. When maintained constantly at −18 C or below, the product can be stored up to 12 months.

A unit of plasma from which the cryoprecipitate has been removed is called single donor plasma (cryoprecipitate removed). Except for the lack of Factor VIII and the loss of 30% to 40% of the fibrinogen originally present in the plasma, this product is the equivalent of single donor plasma and is used for the same purposes.

Single donor plasma is suitable to administer to massive transfusion patients when only red cells, as opposed to whole blood, is available. Such patients may require colloid solution to maintain their intravascular blood volume. The severely traumatized patient receiving large quantities of blood also may derive benefit from single donor plasma. Burn patients, a special category of traumatized patients, often require treatment with large quantities of protein, which can be supplied by the infusion of single donor plasma. Such treatment is not initiated until 24 hours after the injury is sustained.

It must be emphasized that single donor plasma, whether or not previously frozen, has the same hepatitis risk as a unit of blood. Because of this hepatitis risk, the product must never be administered casually to a patient for whom a simple crystalloid solution would suffice.

Single donor plasma, preferably obtained by plasmapheresis of the same donor, is also commonly transfused to hypogammaglobulinemic patients as a source of immunoglobulins.

In the event that a patient sustains massive acute hemorrhage and is transfused with large quantities of blood deficient in the labile coagulation factors, a portion of the administered plasma should be fresh single donor plasma or single donor fresh frozen plasma. This will compensate for the dilutional lowering of his endogenous labile plasma clotting factors caused by the infusion of the stored blood. It is recommended that one unit of single donor fresh frozen plasma be given routinely after ten units of stored blood have been administered. An additional unit of fresh frozen plasma should then be given for each additional five units of blood (see Chapter 6).

Patients who have suffered severe trauma or who have undergone extracorporeal circulation often manifest a coagulopathy due, in part, to consumption of Factors V and VIII, and may require transfusion with fresh frozen plasma. A bleeding patient with disseminated intravascular coagulation (DIC), whatever the etiologic mechanism, may derive benefit from transfusion with fresh frozen plasma, which serves as a source of the labile plasma coagulation factors and fibrinogen. Platelet concentrates may also be transfused in addition to fresh frozen plasma in these clinical situations, or the plasma infused with the platelet concentrates may serve as an adequate substitute for fresh frozen plasma. On the other hand, transfusion of platelets and coagulation factors in DIC may add fuel to the fire.

All single donor plasma products are administered intravenously through a filter. Although no crossmatch is required before transfusion, only ABO group-compatible plasma may be administered to patients. Single donor plasma and single donor fresh frozen plasma, like all other intravenous fluids, can induce fluid overload if given in excess.

If a plasma product is being transfused to correct a clotting deficiency, the therapeutic effectiveness of the product should be monitored periodically.

Albumin

Albumin is a relatively small protein with a molecular weight of 65,000, which accounts for most of the plasma oncotic pressure. Despite the high net negative charge, albumin easily and reversibly binds both cations and anions. This binding affinity makes albumin the primary protein in plasma responsible for binding and transporting or inactivating a host of substances, including drugs, dyes, hormones, metal ions, fatty acids, enzymes, bilirubin, and other metabolites.

Produced in the liver, albumin's half-life in plasma is approximately 20 days. Although daily production is usually quite constant in healthy individuals, diverse factors, including nutrition, hormones, and disease, can significantly influence synthesis. Also, the infusion of dextran or gamma globulin, or the increased synthesis of gamma globulin caused by hyperimmunization results in a prompt depression of albumin synthesis. The site and degradation of albumin is not known.

Albumin (human) is a chemically processed fraction of pooled plasma that has been heat-treated to inactivate the hepatitis virus. It is available as either a 5% buffered saline solution or as a 25% "salt poor" solution. It contains no coagulation components or blood group antigens and can be administered without typing or crossmatching. Plasma protein fraction (PPF) is a similar preparation that contains alpha and beta globulins, as well as albumin. Because of its colloid oncotic effect, administration of 25 gm of albumin will result in a transient blood volume increase of 425 ml.

Used in acute hemorrhagic shock as an oncotic agent, albumin transiently increases the intravascular volume and cardiac output. It is often given in conjunction with crystalloid solutions, which restore coexisting extracellular fluid deficits. Crystalloid solutions alone may be equally effective in treating shock in healthy and relatively young patients. However, in older patients and in those with other medical complications, eg, renal failure, sepsis, or respiratory failure, albumin may be needed to prevent serious hypoalbuminemia.

Albumin is necessary in the treatment of extensive thermal injury because of an increase in permeability of the vascular bed at the site of injury. During the first 24 hours after injury, large volumes of crystalloid solution are required to correct extracellular fluid losses resulting from leakage into the intracellular compartment, while smaller amounts of albumin are required to maintain an adequate intravascular volume. After 24 hours, large amounts of albumin and lesser amounts of crystalloid are required. The need for chronic albumin therapy is determined by continued loss of protein from renal excretion and from denuded areas of skin, and by decreased hepatic albumin synthesis. Albumin should not be used as a nutritional source, but only to correct plasma albumin levels to the extent necessary to maintain an adequate intravascular volume.

Another use for albumin is in the treatment of respiratory distress syndrome, which may develop in patients after shock, trauma, sepsis, and other major medical and surgical disorders. Such patients manifest an increased alveolar-arterial oxygen gradient, secondary to right-to-left shunting of blood, through regions of the lung that are not ventilated, due to pulmonary edema, atelectasis or pneumonia. The primary objective in treatment is the monitoring of fluid intake and output and the administration of diuretics in order to prevent net positive fluid balance. Albumin is used to maintain an effective intravascular volume, since these patients are frequently hypoalbuminemic and, because of diuretic therapy, often develop a low cardiac output. It is necessary to avoid excessive administration of albumin in these patients, whose hemodynamic status is uncertain. Albumin overdose may elevate left arterial pressure, thus aggravating the pulmonary edema. Excessive administration may be prevented by carefully monitoring the patient's central venous or left ventricular filling pressures, and/or other clinical parameters, such as gas exchange and general physical status.

Albumin is often used in conjunction with crystalloid solutions as a pump prime during open-heart surgery, reducing the need for homologous blood transfusions. Albumin is also frequently used during hemodialysis to prevent the transient reduction in intravascular volume and blood pressure, which occurs as a result of removal of fluid. In addition, 25% albumin has been used in the treatment and prevention of cerebral edema.[1]

Other acute situations in which albumin therapy may be indicated include: acute liver failure; resuspension of red cells in albumin during exchange transfusion; replacement of albumin lost as a result of excessive removal of ascites; and occasionally to "prime" or induce diuresis in patients who, due to nephrosis, are severely hypoalbuminemic. However, sustained administration of albumin to patients with chronic liver diseases and nephrosis has not been shown to be of value. Similarly, albumin should not be given as a source of nutrition to chronically debilitated patients. The daily protein requirement of 70 gm is almost unattainable by transfusion of albumin.

Plasma Protein Fraction[2,3]

When intravascular volume expansion is desired and dehydration exists, 5% albumin or Plasma Protein Fraction (PPF) should be used. In situations where extracellular fluid accumulations are being mobilized, 25% "salt poor" albumin is indicated. Since blood volume expansion will occur as quickly as 15 minutes after infusion, 25% albumin should be administered cautiously and should be carefully monitored to prevent acute heart failure or pulmonary edema. Such plasma volume expansion will frequently reduce the hemoglobin concentration and reveal an underlying deficit in red cell mass. In these situations, whole blood can correct the volume and protein deficits more economically, and, therefore, should be administered, rather than packed cells and albumin.

PPF has been reported to contain one or more substances that cause hypotension and even cardiovascular collapse.[5] A few cases of hepatitis have been reported, and one outbreak of hepatitis B was attributed to a manufacturing accident[3]; however, no conclusions can be drawn yet.

Immune Serum Globulin

Immune globulin products are 10% to 16% concentrates of gamma-globulin prepared by cold ethanol fractionation of pooled human plasma. Immune serum globulin (ISG) may be likened to a broad spectrum product, since it is prepared from unselected plasma units from a large number of donors. The major indications for use of this product are passive immunization against viral hepatitis, type A, and immunoglobulin replacement therapy for patients with congenital or acquired immuno-globluin deficiency. A number of specific immune globulin preparations have been manufactured from selected donors' plasma and are used in passive immunizations against infectious diseases, eg, tetanus, rabies, vaccinia, measles, polio, and varicella, and to prevent isoimmunization of Rh-negative mothers bearing Rh-positive infants.

Hepatitis A

ISG should be given as soon as possible after close exposure to a hepatitis A contact, ie, within a household. After exposure to type A carriers in schools, offices, factories or hospitals, ISG is not recommended unless the contact is as intimate as between household members. ISG is also indicated for individuals exposed to blood or serum from a type A hepatitis carrier, due to accidental inoculation. Often recommended as prophylaxis against type A hepatitis, ISG is used in individuals exposed to a common source of hepatitis-A contaminated food or water, individuals in contact with newly imported primates (particularly chimpanzees), and overseas travelers who visit areas where hepatitis A is endemic. The recommended doses for ISG prophylaxis against hepatitis A are 0.5 ml for persons weighing less than 50 lbs; 1.0 ml for persons weighing between 50 and 100 lbs; and 2.0 ml for persons weighing over 100 lbs.

Measles

ISG is also indicated for persons exposed to measles who are known or presumed to be susceptible and who have been exposed within 48 hours before treatment. Such treatment is designed to prevent or modify the clinical manifestations of measles virus infection. These individuals should be given live measles vaccine approximately three months later.

Immunoglobulin Deficiencies

ISG is considered appropriate prophylactic treatment for patients with laboratory-documented immunoglobulin deficiencies. In the absence of an immunoglobulin deficiency state, ISG is not indicated in recurrent respiratory infections or "failure to thrive" syndromes.

Vaccinia

Vaccinia immune globulin (VIG) is recommended therapy for generalized vaccinia, eczema vaccination, or autoinoculation vaccinia, particularly involving the eye, VIG has not been shown to be effective for treating postvaccinial encephalitis.

Rabies

Hyperimmune serum has been shown to be an effective prophylaxis against rabies. In documented rabies exposure, rabies immune globulin should be administered in combination with rabies vaccine in order to provide passive-active protection.

Tetanus

Tetanus immune globulin (TIG) is considered of significant prophylactic value in susceptible individuals exposed to tetanus. It should be given in conujnction with initiation of active immunization with tetanus toxoid.

Varicella

Varicella-Zoster immune globulin (ZIG) is an investigational product distributed by the Center for Disease Control for prevention of varicella in susceptible individuals who have had close exposure (such as household contact) to varicella. The effectiveness of ZIG in high-risk patients who have lymphoproliferative diseases or who are on immunosuppression therapy has not yet been clearly defined.

$Rh_o(D)$ Immune Globulin (RhIG)

RhIG is used to prevent active immunization of Rh-negative individuals against D-positive red blood cells by the principle of antibody-mediated immunosuppression. Active $Rh_o(D)$ antibody formation by Rh-negative women causes Rh hemolytic disease of the newborn in subsequent pregnancies when the fetus is Rh-positive. When the formation of $Rh_o(D)$ antibody is prevented by RhIG, Rh hemolytic disease has not been observed in the subsequent pregnancy.

Indications for RhIG occur following full-term delivery, abortion, and accidental transfusion of Rh-positive blood into Rh-negative individuals. RhIG should be administered to $Rh_o(D)$- or D^u-negative women within 72 hours of the birth of an $Rh_o(D)$- or D^u-positive baby. In addition, RhIG should be administered to such women within 72 hours of a miscarriage, abortion, or ectopic pregnancy, unless the father and/or fetus is known to be $Rh_o(D)$- and D^u-negative.

Prior to administration, the individual must be shown to be $Rh_o(D)$- and D^u-negative. The dose should be calculated to suppress the immune response to the quantity of Rh-positive red cells infused. Calculation of the dose under these circumstances should be based on measurement of the magnitude of the Rh-positive cell infusion, either directly or by a laboratory method, eg, the acid-elution test of Kleihauer-Betke.

RhIG should *not* be administered to an $Rh_o(D)$-positive or D^u-positive individual nor to an $Rh_o(D)$-negative individual who has been actively immunized to the $Rh_o(D)$ antigen by a previous pregnancy or blood transfusion accident.

Hepatitis B

Hepatitis B immune globulin should be given as soon as possible to persons who are exposed to hepatitis B virus by accidental inoculation with contaminated blood or accidental ingestion or splash with HBsAG-positive blood. The dose is 0.05-0.07 ml/kg of body weight, which comes to 3 ml to 5 ml for adults weighing 60 kg to 90 kg. A second identical dose should be administered 25 to 30 days after the exposure episode.

Hepatitis B immune globulin is not necessary for persons who have anti-HBs at the time of exposure since they have been shown to be well protected against hepatitis B from this kind of exposure. It is neither harmful nor beneficial for persons who are HBsAG carriers.

There are a number of other circumstances where hepatitis B immune globulin may be considered. In the case of certain high risk environments, such as renal dialysis units, preventive hygienic measures have proven highly effective in controlling the spread of hepatitis B. In other situations, such as newborn infants whose mothers have acute or chronic hepatitis or spouses and other family members of acutely and chronically infected persons, there are not sufficient data to establish whether hepatitis B immune globulin would be effective, and its use is not recommended at this time.

107

Adverse Reactions

Routine administration of immune globulins is by the intramuscular route. Intravenous administration of the intramuscular preparation is contraindicated because of the risk of severe systemic reactions, including anaphylaxis. Intramuscular administration of any of the immune globulins is frequently associated with local swelling, pain and tenderness, and occasionally with systemic reactions, including rashes, fever, and malaise. Immune globulins prepared by the Cohn cold ethanol fractionation method appear to be essentially devoid of any risk of transmitting viral hepatitis, despite the fact that pooled plasma from large numbers of donors generally is used to manufacture these products.

References

1. Gates EM, Craig W McK: The use of serum albumin in cases of cerebral edema; preliminary report. *Mayo Clin Proc* 23:89, 1948.
2. Tullis JL: Albumin: 2. Guidelines for clinical use. *JAMA* 237: 460-463, 1977.
3. Sgouris JT, Rene A (eds): *Proceedings of the Workshop on Albumin,* (NIH) 76-9265 Government Printing Office, 1975.
4. Skillman JJ, Bipinchandra MP, Tanenbaum BJ: Pulmonary arterio-venous admixture. *Am J Surg* 119:440, 1970.
5. Bland JH, Laver MB, Lowenstein E: Vasodilator effect of commercial 5% plasma protein fraction solutions. *JAMA* 224:1721, 1973.

Chapter 12

TRANSFUSION THERAPY FOR PATIENTS WITH COAGULATION DISORDERS

Dennis Goldfinger, MD, and Anthony F. H. Britten, MD

Congenital Coagulation Disorders

Hemophilia A (Factor VIII Deficiency)

PATIENTS WITH HEMOPHILIA A may require transfusion therapy either on a prophylactic basis, for treatment of established hemorrhage, or in preparation for surgical procedures. Factor VIII can be supplied by transfusion of fresh frozen plasma, cryoprecipitate, or lyophilized Factor VIII concentrate. While fresh frozen plasma contains Factor VIII, this product is not very useful for hemophiliacs, because the volume required to supply enough Factor VIII for treatment usually will result in circulatory overload. Therefore, concentrated preparations of Factor VIII are almost always needed.

The most important complication in transfusing any of these blood products is the possibility of inducing posttransfusion hepatitis. The risk of hepatitis from a single unit of cryoprecipitate is thought to be equal to the risk from a single unit of blood. The more units of cryoprecipitate transfused, the greater the likelihood of transmitting hepatitis. The hepatitis risk from the commercial concentrates of Factor VIII is considerably greater because these products are prepared from pooled plasma obtained from hundreds or thousands of donors. However, most severe hemophiliacs are exposed to large numbers of transfusions during their lifetime and almost invariably will be exposed to hepatitis regardless of the preparations used in their treatment. Therefore, pooled Factor VIII concentrates are both acceptable and useful modes of therapy for these patients. On the other hand, when treating patients with mild hemophilia who may not have been exposed to multiple blood transfusions, cryoprecipitate may be the product of choice.

Numerous studies have demonstrated that patients with severe hemophilia, because of their heavy exposure to blood products, are often carriers of hepatitis B surface antigen (HBsAg). Previously, it had been believed that this carrier state was often a benign condition and, furthermore, that exposure to hepatitis B virus was an inevitable consequence of their disease. Recent studies, however, have demonstrated an alarm-

109

ingly high incidence of severe chronic liver disease in patients with hemophilia.[1,2] Such disease may be the result of hepatitis B virus infection or infection by non-A, non-B hepatitis viruses. Current technology conceivably could prevent exposure to unduly high numbers of donors (eg, by preparation of Factor VIII concentrate from plasma obtained by plasmapheresis of small pools of donors). Whether this approach would significantly reduce the incidence of chronic liver disease in hemophiliacs is not known. The current high prevalence of chronic liver disease in these patients may encourage such studies.

The Factor VIII level considered necessary for adequate hemostasis depends on the kind of bleeding being treated. For minor bleeding and for initial home therapy, a dose calculated to raise the patient's level to 30% to 50% may be used (the 100% level is one unit of Factor VIII per ml of plasma). For major complications, a dose that will raise the level to 50% to 100% should be given. For surgical procedures, a preoperative dose to raise the level to 80% to 100%, followed by postoperative maintenance calculated to keep the level constantly above 50% for two weeks, is recommended.[3-7]

The dose of Factor VIII to be administered may be calculated from the formula in Table 1. When using cryoprecipitate, the Factor VIII levels achieved from a calculated dose will vary, because each cryoprecipitate is prepared from a different donor unit of blood, and the total Factor VIII levels in each cryoprecipitate will differ. Current standards require that a single donor cryoprecipitate should contain a minimum of 80 Factor VIII units per container. An advantage of the commercially-prepared, pooled material is that it is preassayed for its Factor VIII content, and provides a more accurate prediction of posttransfusion levels of Factor VIII.

Table 1.—Calculation of Dosage of Antihemophilic Factor

Calculate Dosage of Factor VIII from the following formula:

$$D = (F - I) \times PV$$

where:

D = Dose of AHF to be administered
(In AHF units)
F = Final desired Factor VIII
concentration
(in AHF units per ml)
I = Initial Factor VIII concentration
(in AHF units per ml)
PV = Plasma Volume
(in milliliters)

When Factor VIII or other coagulation factors initially are infused into a deficient recipient, the recovery of these factors is decreased considerably from what would be expected on the basis of simple dilution in the patient's plasma. Presumably, this is the result of diffusion of the factors into the extravascular space and adherence of factors to various cell surfaces. These recoveries differ widely for each of the various coagulation factors, and it is this consideration that determines the need for, and the size of, the "loading dose" of therapeutic material.

In addition to providing acute therapy at the time of injury or surgery, it is necessary to maintain elevated Factor VIII levels for approximately 10 to 14 days afterward, until enough healing has taken place to prevent subsequent hemorrhage. In considering the dosages that will be necessary to maintain Factor VIII levels in a safe range, frequent Factor VIII assays on the patient's plasma should be performed, and determination of subsequent doses of Factor VIII should be based on these assays. The actual quantitation of Factor VIII levels in the plasma is considered preferable to the use of the partial thromboplastin time in determining the need for, and the quantity of, Factor VIII to be transfused.[6] The in vivo biologic half-life and the required hemostatic level of a particular coagulation factor are the main determinants for the frequency and size of the maintenance doses of therapeutic material. Table 2 shows recommended Factor VIII dosage schedules in hemophilic patients.

In hemophilia A, Factor VIII therapy is most successful when given as soon as possible after trauma or spontaneous bleeding has occurred. This realization has led to the development of home treatment programs for patients with this disease. The development of such programs represents a major advance in hemophilia therapy. Patients are taught to administer Factor VIII preparations to themselves, at home, if any injury or spontaneous hemorrhage should occur.[8,9] Both cryoprecipitate and lyophilized Factor VIII concentrate have been used in these programs.

It has been demonstrated that epsilon aminocaproic acid (EACA) administration can, by preventing normal clot lysis, reduce the dosage of Factor VIII required to maintain hemostasis.[10] EACA has been useful in the treatment of bleeding from the mouth (eg, tooth extraction, torn frenulum) and in major surgery, but should not be used in patients with hematuria, since it may result in blockage of the renal excretory pathway.[6]

von Willebrand's Disease

Study of the mechanisms leading to the hemostatic defects in patients with von Willebrand's disease is currently an area of intense interest in the field of hemostasis. It appears that these patients have two major coagu-

Table 2.—Replacement Therapy in Hemophilia A and B and von Willebrand's Disease

Hemostatic Level (% of Normal)	Therapeutic Material	MINOR BLEEDING Uncomplicated hemarthroses; Hematomas in noncritical areas; Dressing changes; Arthrocentesis; Removal of sutures and drains, etc. Single Dose	MAJOR BLEEDING Hematomas in critical locations; Head injuries; Traumatic injuries; Tooth extractions; Major surgery Loading Dose	Maintenance Dose (approximate)
HEMOPHILIA A (Factor VIII Deficiency) 30 - 50	Cryo-precipitate	1.25-1.75 bags/10 kg	5 bags/10 kg	1.75 bags/10 kg every 8 hr for 1-2 days; every 12 hr thereafter
	Factor VIII Concentrate	12-20 units/kg	40 units/kg	10-15 units/kg every 8 hr for 1-2 days; every 12 hr thereafter

Condition		Component			
HEMOPHILIA B (Factor IX Deficiency)	15 - 25	Plasma	15-20 ml/kg; may be necessary to repeat dose every 8-12 hr up to 4-5 additional doses		Generally ineffective.
		Factor IX Concentrate	Generally not required	Single dose calculated to raise level to 100%	Follow loading dose in 4-6 hr with dose to maintain patient above 35%. Continue to maintain level above 35% by doses every 12-24 hr
von WILLEBRAND'S DISEASE	30 - 50	Plasma	10 ml/kg		10 ml/kg every 8-12 hr for 1-2 days. Lesser amounts (depending on clinical status) thereafter
		Cryo-precipitate			1 bag/10 kg every 8-12 hr for 1-2 days. Lesser amounts (if clinically indicated) thereafter

113

lation abnormalities, both related to functions of the Factor VIII molecule. First, the patient may be deficient in Factor VIII procoagulant activity to such a magnitude as to impair hemostasis. A second deficiency, that of a factor responsible for normal platelet activity, may result in impairment of platelet hemostatic function.

Patients with von Willebrand's disease should be treated with administration of Factor VIII to provide hemostatically effective procoagulant and platelet functional levels. Treatment of these patients should take into account the following considerations:

1. The factor affecting platelet function is present in both fresh frozen plasma and cryoprecipitate, but is not contained in most commercially prepared Factor VIII concentrates[11,12]; therefore, such concentrates should not be used to treat these patients.

2. The rise in Factor VIII procoagulant concentration, following administration of cryoprecipitate or plasma, is sustained much longer in von Willebrand's disease than in hemophilia A; therefore, when treating these patients, transfusions need to be given less frequently.

3. Platelet transfusion has no place in the treatment of von Willebrand's disease, since the patient's platelets are not intrinsically defective. Transfused platelets function abnormally in the plasma of patients with von Willebrand's disease.

4. Careful clinical monitoring is essential for determining the course of therapy for patients with this disease. While this is true in the treatment of all coagulopathies, it is especially so in von Willebrand's disease, because laboratory tests used to monitor hemostatic function do not necessarily reflect the clinical status of the patient. Factor VIII procoagulant concentration can be measured, as in the management of hemophilia A. However, this determination does not necessarily correlate with the level of platelet hemostatic activity. Tests of platelet function, including the template bleeding time and measurements of ristocetin aggregation, can be used to monitor the need for Factor VIII administration, but these tests do not necesssarily correlate with clinical hemostasis in the patient.

Hemophilia B (Factor IX Deficiency)

Patients with hemophilia B may require transfusion therapy to supply hemostatic levels of Factor IX during episodes of traumatic or spontaneous bleeding, or in conjunction with surgery. Adequate levels of Factor IX can be supplied sometimes with fresh frozen plasma or

114

cryoprecipitate-depleted plasma, but concentrated Factor IX preparations usually are needed in order to achieve satisfactorily high levels of Factor IX in patients with severe deficiency. As with Factor VIII replacement, therapy with Factor IX-containing material should be continued for approximately 10 to 14 days, until adequate healing has taken place. Factor IX concentrations above 25% should be maintained during this period. Since the half-life of Factor IX is longer than that of Factor VIII, adequate levels can be achieved by infusions of Factor IX-containing material every 12 to 24 hours. On the other hand, the initial loss of plasma activity (extravascular distribution plus adherence to cell surfaces) is greater for Factor IX than for Factor VIII, so that a considerably larger loading dose is needed in treating patients with hemophilia B. (See Table 2 for recommended dosage.)

Factor IX concentrate (prothrombin complex concentrate) is a commercial preparation containing high levels of the vitamin K dependent factors—Factors II (prothrombin), VII, IX and X. The use of Factor IX concentrate carries two potential hazards. First, there is a high risk of hepatitis, since this product is prepared from large pools of donor plasma. Second, there have been several reports of increased intravascular coagulation, with a tendency to thrombosis, in patients receiving prothrombin complex.[13] This was thought to be due to the presence of activated coagulation factors in these preparations. However, recent studies with new lots of Factor IX concentrate have failed to demonstrate the presence of activated coagulation factors,[14] and have demonstrated no evidence of thrombotic complications. While the hazards of Factor IX concentrate must be weighed against the potential benefits of the product to the patient, for patients with severe hemophilia B, Factor IX concentrate may be the only satisfactory product for supplying hemostatically effective levels of Factor IX.

Factor XI Deficiency

Patients with Factor XI deficiency usually do not have clinical bleeding manifestations of the magnitude seen in patients with severe hemophilia A or B. In some patients, however, there may be significant and dangerous bleeding, especially at times of major trauma or surgery. No concentrated Factor XI preparation is available for transfusion, but such a product probably is not needed since adequate hemostatis generally can be achieved with the use of fresh frozen plasma or cryoprecipitate-poor plasma. Adequate hemostatic levels of 30% to 50% usually can be maintained easily, because of the relatively long half-life of Factor XI. A preoperative dose of fresh frozen plasma of 10 ml/kg, followed by a daily maintenance dose of 5 ml/kg, has been found to be effective for

115

patients undergoing major surgical procedures. As with the treatment of hemophilia, daily dosage of Factor XI should be based on frequent determinations of the Factor XI levels in the patient's plasma.

Deficiencies of Other Coagulation Factors

Deficiencies of fibrinogen, prothrombin, Factor V, Factor VII, Factor X, Factor XII and Factor XIII are very rare disorders. Patients with Factor XII deficiency have no clinical manifestations of increased bleeding, and require no specific replacement therapy, even during major surgical procedures. This also is true of patients deficient in other factors of the contact system, including Fletcher Factor and Fitzgerald Factor. Patients with deficiencies of other coagulation factors may experience significant hemorrhagic complications requiring replacement therapy.[15] Treatment is summarized in Table 3. It should be noted that the treatment of congenital fibrinogen deficiency can be well-managed with the use of cryoprecipitates, which contain concentrated fibrinogen.[16, 17] Commercially-prepared fibrinogen concentrate is no longer available for use in humans because of the unacceptabily high hepatitis risk of this product.[16]

Acquired Coagulation Disorders

Disseminated Intravascular Coagulation

Patients with disseminated intravascular coagulation (DIC) may consume their coagulation factors during the process and develop a subsequent hemorrhagic diathesis. Therefore, in severe DIC from any underlying cause, hemorrhage may become a significant clinical problem. In such cases, replacement therapy with blood products containing the missing coagulation components may be needed. However, it must be noted that the only effective means for treating DIC is to correct the underlying disorder that precipitated intravascular clotting. When the underlying disease cannot be controlled easily, or when the DIC is very severe, anticoagulant therapy with heparin may be used to interrupt the coagulation process. Results of such anticoagulation have not been encouraging, probably because therapy in reported cases has been instituted too late in the course of DIC, or because the underlying disease process leading to DIC could not be managed successfully.

Potentially, any or all coagulation factors and platelets may be consumed during the process of DIC, making replacement transfusion desirable. Platelet concentrates are used to supply platelets, if needed. Fresh frozen plasma may be used as a source of all other blood coagulation

Table 3.–Replacement Therapy for Miscellaneous Hereditary Coagulation Disorders

DISORDER	HEMOSTATIC LEVEL (% of Normal)	THERAPEUTIC MATERIAL	LOADING DOSE	MAINTENANCE DOSE
Fibrinogen Deficiency	10 - 25	Cryoprecipitate	4 bags/10 kg	1 bag/10 kg every other day
Prothrombin Deficiency	20 - 40	Plasma (fresh frozen or cryoprecipitate-poor)	15 ml/kg	5-10 ml/kg daily
		Prothrombin Complex	20 μ/kg	10 μ/kg daily
Factor V Deficiency	15 - 25	Plasma (fresh frozen or cryoprecipitate-poor)	20 ml/kg	10 ml/kg every 12 hours
Factor VII Deficiency	5 - 10	Plasma (fresh frozen or cryoprecipitate-poor)	10 ml/kg	
		Prothrombin Complex	10 μ/kg	Not required (15)
Factor X Deficiency	10 - 20	Plasma (fresh frozen or cryoprecipitate-poor)	15 ml/kg	10 ml/kg daily
		Prothrombin Complex	15 μ/kg	10 μ/kg daily
Factor XI Deficiency	10	Plasma (fresh frozen or cryoprecipitate-poor)	10 ml/kg	5 ml/kg daily
Factor XIII Deficiency	2 - 3	Plasma (fresh frozen or cryoprecipitate-poor)	5 ml/kg every 2-3 weeks	Not required

components, although it may be advantageous to supply certain components in concentrated form. In such cases, the use of cryoprecipitates for the specific replacement of Factor VIII and fibrinogen may be useful.[17] If red cell transfusion is necessary, because of blood loss, the use of fresh whole blood usually is of no special value, since the content of coagulation factors and platelets in fresh whole blood generally is too small to be of help. Therefore, the use of packed or washed red bood cells to supply hemoglobin requirements, combined with fresh frozen plasma, cryoprecipitates and platelet concentrates, as deemed necessary, would seem to be the most logical approach to transfusion therapy in such patients.

Liver Disease

Patients with severe hepatic failure may be unable to manufacture those coagulation factors which are produced by the liver. These include the vitamin K dependent factors (Factors II, VII, IX and X), as well as Factor V and fibrinogen. Such patients may require coagulation component therapy for control of hemorrhage, although management of such patients is often quite difficult. If transfusion of coagulation components is necessary, it should be accomplished with the use of fresh frozen plasma, which contains enough of the liver-dependent factors to achieve adequate hemostatic levels in such patients, and has the advantage of minimizing hepatitis risk. Concentrated prothrombin complex carries a significant hepatitis risk, and its use is contraindicated in liver disease.

Vitamin K may be given to patients with severe liver disease, in an attempt to induce endogenous production of vitamin K dependent factors, but this is of no value in the majority of cases. Patients with severe liver disease frequently may develop disseminated intravascular coagulation and increased fibrinolysis. In such patients, the distinction between DIC and simple underproduction of coagulation factors may be difficult.

Vitamin K Deficiency

Vitamin K deficiency will result in underproduction of four of the coagulation factors produced by the liver—Factors II (prothrombin), VII, IX, and X. Treatment consists of parenteral administration of vitamin K_1 (generally 10 mg intramuscularly or intravenously), so that the patient may synthesize adequate quantities of these coagulation factors. This therapy is usually effective in a matter of hours. Occasionally, it may be necessary to supply the needed coagulation factors more quickly, so that, in addition to vitamin K_1 administration, the infusion of plasma may be useful (500 ml to 1000 ml). The use of prothrombin complex is contraindicated in this situation.

Anticoagulant Overdose

Warfarin (Coumadin, Dicumarol)

Patients with overdoses of warfarin or related compounds may develop a severe hemorrhagic diathesis due to depressed levels of Factors II, VII, IX and X (the vitamin K dependent factors). Treatment consists of preventing further drug ingestion, and possible administration of vitamin K, in order to stimulate endogenous coagulation factor production. If the patient is not bleeding dangerously, the use of a small dose of vitamin K_1 (1 mg intramuscularly or intravenously) should be considered, to prevent the development of a refractory state to further warfarin therapy.[18] If hemorrhage is severe, and more rapid reversal of anti-coagulation is needed, standard doses of vitamin K_1 (10 mg to 20 mg) should be used. It also may be advisable to provide coagulation factors by transfusing plasma. Plasma (either fresh frozen of cryoprecipitate-poor) in a dose of 500 ml to 1000 ml (two to four units) usually will supply sufficient coagulation components to provide adequate hemostasis. Prothrombin complex concentrate, because of its great hepatitis risk, is contraindicated.

Heparin

Bleeding secondary to heparin administration generally requires no treatment other than discontinuation of heparin infusion. If more rapid reversal of heparin effect is needed, protamine sulfate may be administered. Transfusion of coagulation factors is not needed in this situation.

Massive Blood Transfusion

Patients who receive a massive blood transfusion may develop hemorrhagic complications due to a platelet washout effect since the transfused blood may be depleted of viable platelets. This problem is diagnosed by monitoring the platelet count, and platelet concentrates are indicated if the platelet count falls below $50,000/mm^3$.

Washout of plasma coagulation factors has never been clearly documented, although the association of coagulopathies with massive transfusion is sometimes seen. The concomitant presence of disseminated intravascular coagulation should be considered in such cases. The routine use of one unit of fresh frozen plasma for every five units of stored blood has been suggested for patients expected to receive large amounts of blood. However, the need for such therapy has been questioned and has provoked differences of opinion. The decision is, thus, up to the individual physician. The prothrombin time (PT) and partial thromboplastin time (PTT) are a simple, reliable and quick index of the development of any acquired coagulopathy. If the PT is lengthened beyond 18 seconds (control 12), and not due to disseminated intravascular coagulation, fresh frozen plasma may be helpful in correcting the defect. The problems are more complicated if the patient has hepatocellular insufficiency; the prophylactic use of fresh frozen plasma can be rationalized in such cases if the original prothrombin time was prolonged.

Patients receiving a massive transfusion often are administered considerable amounts of citrate, but a significant coagulopathy due to hypocalcemia probably never occurs. Cardiac arrhythmias will occur before calcium levels are lowered sufficiently to affect coagulation.

Optimal transfusion therapy can only be given to massively transfused patients in conjunction with careful laboratory monitoring of the hemostatic status of the patient. A full "coagulogram" may be too time-consuming to be useful in the acute situation, but the platelet count, the partial thromboplastin time and the prothrombin time can quickly give helpful information. The subsequent completion of more detailed studies will aid retrospective evaluation of these complex patients.

Coagulation Factor Inhibitors

Inhibitors to Factor VIII may be seen in patients with hemophilia A, or as an acquired disorder in nonhemophilic individuals. Such patients may develop hemorrhagic complications that can be extremely difficult to manage. The initial attempt to treat such patients should include infusions of massive quantities of Factor VIII preparations (either Factor VIII concentrates or cryoprecipitates). For patients unresponsive to this therapy, immunosuppressive drugs have been utilized, with some reported success.[19] Exchange transfusion or exchange plasmapheresis to remove the inhibitor, followed by infusion of Factor VIII concentrates, may be attempted, and has been demonstrated to be successful in some cases.[20, 21] Concomitant immunosuppressive therapy with azathioprine or cyclophosphamide is usually necessary to prevent rapid reaccumulation of antibody.

Infusions of commercially-prepared Factor IX concentrates, as well as an experimental product—Activated Prothrombin Complex (Hyland Laboratories)—have been used with success in controlling bleeding in such patients.[22] These preparations are effective because they contain activated coagulation factors, which bypass the need for Factor VIII. Recent studies, however, have demonstrated a lack of such activated factors in current lots of Factor IX concentrates,[14, 23] as a result of the manufacturers' efforts to remove these factors from their products. While removal of the activated coagulation factors makes these concentrates

120

safer for patients being treated for Factor IX deficiency, it eliminates their usefulness in managing patients with Factor VIII inhibitors.[23] The experimental Hyland product is still available, however, and is useful for these patients.

Transfusion of Factor VIII-containing blood products to patients with Factor VIII inhibitors often can stimulate increased antibody (inhibitor) production. Such transfusions, therefore, should be reserved for dangerous or life-threatening bleeding episodes. Less severe bleeding should be treated, if possible, without resorting to Factor VIII infusions.

Acquired inhibitors to other coagulation factors are rarely encountered. Often, such inhibitors appear to be active only in vitro and have little clinical significance. The presence of such inhibitors, however, can cause great consternation since there may be no way of ascertaining that the in vitro abnormalities will not be duplicated in vivo. Such patients must be managed on an individual basis and may or may not require transfusion therapy.

References

1. Hasiba UW, Spero JA, Lewis JH: Chronic liver dysfunction in multi-transfused hemophiliacs. *Transfusion* 17:490-494, 1977.
2. Hilgartner MW, Giardina P: Liver dysfunction in patients with hemophilia A, B, and von Willebrand's disease. *Transfusion* 17:495-499, 1977.
3. Wintrobe MM (ed): *Clinical Hematology,* Philadelphia, 1974, pp 1158-1232.
4. Williams WJ, Buetler E, Erslev AJ, et al (eds): *Hematology,* New York, McGraw-Hill, 1977, pp 1561-1576.
5. Schmidt PJ, Grindon AJ: Blood and blood components in the prevention and control of bleeding. *JAMA* 202:967-969, 1976.
6. Kasper CK: Personal Communication.
7. Biggs R (ed): *Human Blood Coagulation, Haemostasis and Thrombosis.* Oxford, Blackwell Scientific Publications, 1972.
8. Levine PH: Efficacy of self-therapy in hemophilia. *N Engl J Med* 291:1381-1384, 1974.
9. Rabiner SF, Telfer MD: Home transfusion for patients with hemophilia A. *N Engl J Med* 283:1011-1015, 1970.
10. Storti E, Ascari E, Molinari E, et al: Saving of cryoprecipitate in the surgery of hemophilic patients. *N Engl J Med* 287:198-199, 1972.
11. Perkins HA: Correction of the hemostatic defects in von Willebrand's disease. *Blood* 30:375, 1967.
12. Green D, Potter EV: Failure of AHF concentrate to control bleeding in von Willebrand's disease. *Am J Med* 60:357-360, 1976.

13. Kasper CK: Postoperative thromboses in hemophilia B. *N Engl J Med* 289:160, 1976.
14. Penner JA, Leach K, Rohwedder J: Thrombogenic characteristics of activated and standard concentrates of prothrombin complex. *Clin Res* 24:572A, 1976.
15. Britten AFH, Salzman E: Surgery in congenital disorders of blood coagulation. *Surg Gynecol Obstet* 123:1333-1358, 1966.
16. Bove JR: Fibrinogen—is the benefit worth the risk? *Transfusion* 18:129-136, 1978.
17. Hattersley PG, Kunkel M: Cryoprecipitates as a source of fibrinogen in treatment of disseminated intravascular coagulation (DIC). *Transfusion* 16:641-645, 1976.
18. Deykin D: Warfarin therapy. *N Engl J Med* 283:691-694, 801-803, 1970.
19. Hultin MB, Shapiro SS, Bowman HS, et al: Immunosuppressive therapy for Factor VIII inhibitors. *Blood* 48:95-108, 1976.
20. Strauss HS: Acquired circulatory anticoagulants in hemophilia A. *N Engl J Med* 281:866-873, 1969.
21. McCullough J, Fortuny IE, Kennedy BJ, et al: Rapid plasma exchange with continuous flow centrifuge. *Transfusion* 13:94-99, 1973.
22. Kurczynski EM, Penner JA: Activated prothrombin concentrate for patients with Factor VIII inhibitors. *N Engl J Med* 291:164-167, 1974.
23. Penner JA, Abildgaard CF: Ineffectiveness of certain prothrombin complex concentrates in treatment of patients with inhibitors of Factors VIII and IX. *N Engl J Med* 300:565-566, 1979.

Chapter 13

PERINATAL, NEONATAL, AND EXCHANGE TRANSFUSIONS

Julian B. Schorr, MD

Introduction

THIS CHAPTER deals primarily with transfusion therapy during the first year of life, because the unique aspects of pediatric transfusions are largely confined to infancy. Beyond one year of age, the differences which distinguish pediatric from adult transfusions relate almost entirely to the size of the patient.

Among the unique features which characterize transfusion in infancy are the reasons for transfusion, which may include the presence of a disease acquired in utero or a congenital disorder often fatal in childhood. Other differences relate to blood volume in small babies, the hemoglobin levels, and hemoglobin configuration peculiar to infancy. Also, the routes for transfusing babies may utilize blood vessels not ordinarily available in adults, or injection sites other than blood vessels. Lastly, the risk of blood-transmitted infection may be enhanced by the increased susceptibility of the immunologically immature neonate.[1] In evaluating the need for transfusing an infant, it is necessary to consider the specific aspects of pediatric transfusions.[2]

Blood Volume

Blood volume in the newborn infant is relatively larger than in the older child and adult. There is also greater variation in the normal figures. Premature infants have blood volumes of 90 to 105 ml/kg; in full-term infants, blood volumes cluster between 83 and 95 ml/kg. These elevations of blood volume norms are short-lived, and by two or three months of age, blood volume of healthy infants approaches the 72 to 74 ml/kg of healthy adults.

Hemoglobin and Hematocrit Values

Hemoglobin levels in newborns cannot be evaluated accurately without knowing the source of the blood specimen. The concentration of cord blood hemoglobin is lower than simultaneous venous blood hemoglobin, which in turn is lower than capillary hemoglobin, as noted below:

123

Cord Blood (16.8 gm/dl) is 10% less than Venous Blood (18.5 gm/dl) is 10% less than Capillary Blood (20.3 gm/dl)

Because of efflux of plasma water from the circulation during the first day, hemoglobin and hematocrit levels rise so that at 24 hours of age, venous levels average 19 gm/dl, and 61%, respectively.

After increasing over the first six hours of life, the differences between venous and capillary hemoglobin levels remain stable for three days, then gradually disappear by the sixth day. These differences can be decreased, but not eliminated, by warming the skin prior to capillary blood collection.

In premature infants, initial hemoglobin and hematocrit values are lower than in full-term infants, and depend on the gestational age. Infants born prior to 34 weeks of gestation demonstrate sex differences in hemoglobin of approximately the same degree as seen between men and women.[3]

During the first three months of life, hemoglobin levels of full-term infants decrease progressively, usually leveling at 11 gm/dl. When a term infant's hemoglobin falls below 10.5 gm/dl, evaluation of the anemia is indicated.

In healthy infants born prematurely, levels as low as 8.5 gm/dl are common, and the nadir usually is reached between five and eight weeks of age. If adequate iron is provided, the hemoglobin will rise, reaching levels of about 11 gm/dl by the fifth month. At one time, premature infants were transfused regularly; today, if repeated venesection for blood studies does not accentuate this "physiological anemia," transfusion rarely is necessary.

Fetal Hemoglobin

Hemoglobin F, which predominates in infants, has an increased affinity for oxygen, the P_{50} being six to eight mm Hg below that of hemoglobin A. Thus, at physiological oxygen tensions, less oxygen will be released to the tissues. The cause of this increased oxygen affinity is that 2, 3-DPG is bound to HbF to a lesser degree than to HbA. This difference persists for about six months, after which HbF levels fall to below 10% of total hemoglobin, and the effect on the P_{50} becomes undiscernible. The physiologic significance of the increased oxygen affinity of the newborn infant's blood is not known.

Disorders in Infancy Requiring Exchange Transfusion Therapy

Hemolytic Disease of the Newborn (HDN)

Among the disorders of infancy most characteristically associated with exchange transfusion is hemolytic disease of the newborn due to maternal isoimmunization to the Rh factor. While the incidence of this form of HDN has markedly decreased, erythroblastosis remains a significant cause for neonatal morbidity, and laboratory evaluation of the pregnant woman remains a major function of the transfusion service.

Maternal Screening

The objective of prenatal immunohematological testing is to identify those women at risk of having babies affected by HDN. Once identified, such women can be followed in order to predict risk to the fetus, to determine optimal time for delivery, and to coordinate the efforts of the obstetrician, transfusion service medical director, and pediatrician, all to provide optimal care to the affected neonate.

ABO and Rh typing and antibody screening should be performed on the first obstetrical visit. All pregnant women, Rh-positive as well as Rh-negative, should be screened for unexpected antibodies since blood group antibodies other than Anti-D can cause HDN. If the initial antibody screening test is negative, a second antibody screening test should be performed later in the pregnancy (32 to 34 weeks). Obstetricians should be aware of the disadvantages of having maternal antibody screening done at laboratories other than the one where the infant will be crossmatched. This practice can cause delays in confirming the maternal antibody and in finding compatible blood for transfusion at the time of the delivery. If all positive antibody screening tests are reported to the hospital transfusion service, and if follow-up studies in immunized women are then conducted at the hospital, the screening procedures may be done by laboratories away from the hospital.

If the initial antibody screening test is positive, the antibody specificity should be determined and a protocol for further testing of the mother should be established. This protocol should include genotyping of father, antibody titres, and amniocentesis, when indicated.

Paternal Testing

ABO-compatible red cells from the father may be included in the mother's antibody screening test, and may detect the presence of an antibody to a low incidence antigen. Genotyping of the father should also be done when an antibody known to cause HDN is found in the mother. The father's red cells should be tested to determine, if possible, whether he is homozygous or heterozygous for the gene producing the immunizing antigen. This will aid in establishing the probabilities of the baby's blood group and the likelihood of HDN in future pregnancies.

125

Antibodies Associated with HDN

Certain antibodies are more likely to cause HDN than others. IgM antibodies usually do not cross the placenta and, thus, do not cause HDN. Antibodies to antigens incompletely developed at birth, such as Lewis or I, do not cause HDN. Significant antibodies that can cross the placenta and cause HDN are of the IgG class. The most common cause of severe HDN has been anti-D (Rh_o), followed by anti-c, anti-Kell, and anti-E. HDN also may be caused by IgG antibodies produced against antigens in the Duffy, Kidd, MN and other blood group systems; IgG antibodies to low incidence (family) antigens have occasionally been implicated. Today, IgG antibodies in the ABO system are the most frequent cause of HDN. However, no prenatal test is available to accurately predict ABO disease.

Titers

Titers should be performed on all significant antibodies (other than ABO) discovered in a pregnant woman's serum, and should be repeated at intervals during the pregnancy. By performing the titer from a stored frozen serum specimen drawn earlier in the pregnancy and comparing the value with subsequent samples drawn from the patient, it is possible to establish whether the level of antibody is increasing, decreasing, or remaining constant. In the first sensitized pregnancy, a rising titer indicates that the baby will probably be affected with HDN. Serial titers in subsequent pregnancies may have some value, but do not always correlate with the severity of the disease. The principal value of the antibody titer is identification of those women who are candidates for amniocentesis. The transfusion service medical director should assist the obstetrician in determining the necessity of doing further studies, including amniocentesis.

Amniocentesis

If the indirect antiglobulin test titer is 1:32 or greater, (titer values may vary slightly from laboratory to laboratory) or when there is a history of previously affected infants, examination of the amniotic fluid for bilirubin-like pigments should be considered.

The severity of the hemolytic process in utero can be judged by spectrophotometric examination of the amniotic fluid, which undergoes changes in optical density due to the presence of bilirubin-related pigments.

If the results of repeated amniocentesis indicate that the deviation from normal optical density at 450μ is approaching or has entered Liley's Zone III, and the gestational age of the fetus is between 24 weeks and 35 weeks, intrauterine transfusion should be considered.[4] Once intrauterine transfusions are initiated, they are usually repeated at 10-to-4 day intervals until delivery of the infant.

Intrauterine Transfusion (IUT)

Intrauterine blood transfusion (IUT) was first described in 1963 by Dr. A. W. Liley of New Zealand for the treatment of potentially fatal HDN due to maternofetal Rh-incompatibility. With the use of IUT, as many as 60% of babies who would have died of HDN can be saved.[4]

Blood is injected into the peritoneal cavity of the fetus, from which it is readily absorbed into the infant's vascular space. The amount of blood transfused depends on gestational age (see Table 1). The last transfusion is often given at the 34th week, and delivery planned for the 36th week.

Table 1.—Intrauterine Blood Transfusion

Gestational Age (weeks)	Volume of Packed Cells
24	40 ml
26	60 ml
28	80 ml
30	100 ml
32	120 ml
34	120 ml

The infant with HDN delivered before the 36th week may not do well. This is especially true when respiratory distress syndrome (RDS) develops. To determine the likelihood of RDS, the ratio of lecithin to sphingomyelin in the amniotic fluid is determined. If the ratio is greater than 2.5:1, RDS is very unlikely. If that ratio is below 2.5:1, delivery is often postponed and further IUT are given.

For intrauterine transfusion, group O, Rh-negative frozen red cells, or packed red cells less than 72 hours old, tested for compatibility with the mother, should be used. An antibody identification panel is done before each transfusion to make sure that the mother has not developed other unexpected antibodies. If she has, the O Rh-negative blood should also lack these antigens.

Following intrauterine or neonatal transfusion, rare instances of apparent graft-versus-host (GVH) disease have been reported, presumably the result of the transfusion of viable lymphocytes. For this reason, some transfusionists irradiate blood used in perinatal transfusion as well as that used in transfusing immunoincompetent or immunosuppressed patients.[5,6] The recommended doses range from 1,500 to 3,000 rads. Whether the processing of frozen blood sufficiently reduces the number of viable lymphocytes is not known. Telischi et al have reported the presence of immunocompetent lymphocytes in units of frozen deglycerolized blood.[7]

Intrauterine transfusion is not without other hazards—both to the mother and the baby. The placenta can be injured if the needle is not placed within the peritoneal space of the fetus. Also, some women will have spontaneous abortions after the first or second IUT, especially when the transfusion is given early in pregnancy.

After delivery, if the IUTs have been successful, the baby will frequently have a negative direct Coombs test, and the red cells in the infant may be almost entirely group O Rh-negative. The Kleihauer-Betke stain for fetal red blood cells may also show almost all adult cells. Even so, repeated exchange transfusions are often required to combat anemia and rapidly increasing bilirubinemia.

Neonatal Evaluations and Exchange Transfusion for HDN

It seems desirable that a cord blood sample from every newborn be submitted to the transfusion service for ABO and Rh grouping and a direct Coombs test. By adhering to this policy unsuspected cases of HDN will be discovered, permitting prompt treatment when indicated.

Although increasing levels of bilirubinemia constitute the usual laboratory indication for exchange transfusion, criteria have been established for choosing, at birth, the infant with Rh-HDN who should receive an immediate exchange transfusion. In these infants, the presence in the cord blood of a positive direct antiglobulin test, plus a cord hemoglobin below 12 gm/dl and/or a cord bilirubin of greater than 4.5 gm/dl indicates the need for an immediate exchange transfusion.[8]

Infants with HDN not exchange-transfused at birth are followed closely with bilirubin determinations at three- to six-hour intervals to evaluate the level as well as the rate of rise of serum bilirubin.

The critical level of hyperbilirubinemia varies with gestational age and birthweight. For full-term infants, levels about 20 mg/dl are considered potentially dangerous; for premature infants between 1700 gm and 2500 gm, exchange transfusion is recommended at 15 to 17 mg/dl, and in smaller prematures, levels above 12 mg/dl may be dangerous. In treating jaundiced premature infants, other factors, particularly the presence of respiratory distress and acidemia, are important in determining the need for exchange transfusion.

The exchange transfusion in the infant has two major purposes: (1) the treatment of anemia developing from hemolysis caused by maternal alloantibodies; and (2) the reduction in unconjugated bilirubin level which might otherwise cause kernicterus. When HDN is the reason for exchange transfusion, administration of blood negative for the target antigen probably decreases the likelihood of continuing hyper-bilirubinemia.

The recommended exchange transfusion volume equals two infant's blood volumes (180 ml/kg) and achieves a 90% exchange. One unit of whole blood approximates two infant blood volumes, and, therefore, is sufficient for this exchange. When the infant's weight is more than 3.0 kg, calculation of the volume to be used exceeds one unit. However, since a 70% exchange is accomplished with the first blood volume equivalent, the loss of efficiency when large infants are exchanged with 500 ml is negligible and a second unit of blood is rarely necessary.

The selected blood should be no more than five days old. CPD anti-coagulant is preferred over ACD because of its higher pH, its better preservation of 2,3-DPG, and its decreased levels of potassium and citrate. Heparin is preferred by some as an anticoagulant, although it has been shown to increase the plasma concentration of free fatty acids which can compete with bilirubin for albumin binding sites.[9] No clear advantage of heparinized blood has been demonstrated and the problems associated with its short shelf-life have limited its use. Frozen red cells represent an excellent product for neonatal exchange transfusion, particularly when blood less than five days old is unavailable. ABO-compatible fresh frozen plasma provides an excellent medium for resuspension of frozen red cells.

Albumin may be added to the blood to increase the infant's bilirubin binding capacity.[8] Approximately 30 ml to 50 ml of 25% albumin is added to a unit of whole blood from which 60 ml to 90 ml of supernatant plasma have been removed. Although addition of albumin might be expected to increase posttransfusion "bilirubin rebound," there is little evidence that this occurs. Thus, the anxiety that albumin administration may confuse subsequent evaluation of jaundiced infants appears inappropriate. In Rh-HDN, the blood used should be Rh_o-negative. When mother and baby are of the same ABO groups, group-specific blood can be used. If they are of different ABO groups, group-O blood, or group-O cells resuspended in plasma compatible with the infant is recommended. This permits crossmatching with the mother's serum. When the mother's serum is available, it should be crossmatched with blood for the initial transfusion. When the mother's blood is not available, crossmatching with the infant's serum is adequate. The admonition that the mother's serum *must* be used in the crossmatch is not valid; only an antibody that is detectable in the infant's serum or red cell eluate can cause significant hemolysis.

For ABO HDN, Rh-specific group-O blood or group-O cells in plasma compatible with the infant may be used. On the rare occasion when the

129

maternal serum contains an antibody to a high incidence antigen and no compatible blood is available, the mother's red cells may be used, resuspended in plasma compatible with the infant's ABO group.

The temperature of the blood is important because newborn infants become hypothermic when given cold blood. Blood should be placed in a warming device, preferably one that is "in-line" to raise the temperature of the blood to 35 C to 37 C during administration (see Chapter 3).

Disseminated Intravascular Coagulopathy

Although exchange transfusion is usually performed in jaundiced infants with HDN, occasional exchange transfusions are performed for neonatal jaundice associated with hereditary spherocytosis, enclosed hemorrhage, infantile pyknocytosis, or infection. Recently, several other indications for exchange transfusion have been suggested and, as Rh-immune disease has decreased, they have become increasingly important. One of these is disseminated intravascular coagulopathy (DIC).

DIC results in a hemorrhagic state leading to depletion of platelets and diverse coagulation factors, including fibrinogen, with the production of fibrin split products. Conditions under which DIC is seen include sepsis and RDS. The frequency with which this disorder is diagnosed varies from one neonatal care unit to the next, because there is no precise definition of DIC in the neonate. In 1975, Hathaway[10] noted that "four types of intravascular coagulation syndromes may be recognized in the newborn period." Evaluation of DIC in the neonate is difficult, and the infant's normal tendency to deficiencies of Factors II, VII, XI, and X clouds the laboratory diagnosis.

There are distinct differences of opinion regarding optimal therapy of DIC. Eliminating the underlying cause is of paramount importance. Beyond that, there are advocates of heparinization, with or without use of platelets and fresh plasma transfusions. Exchange transfusion has also been employed in this condition. The process serves to replace coagulation factors and clear the body of fibrin degradation products that might inhibit coagulation.[10] The results have appeared promising and an increasing number of exchanges are being performed for this condition.

Whether the use of blood less than 48 hours old for the purpose of exchanging HbA for HbF in neonates with RDS will prove a valuable addition to the therapy of this disorder is, at present, a moot point, although Delivoria-Papadopoulos et al have described encouraging results.[11]

Route of Exchange Transfusion

The umbilical vein remains the simplest and probably the safest route for neonatal exchange transfusions, and excellent disposable exchange transfusion equipment is available. The umbilical artery may also be used and is frequently catheterized for prolonged periods of parenteral alimentation in premature infants. Although complete asepsis is not possible when the umbilical stump is employed as a port of entry, the use of a surgical prep, and of sterile gloves and equipment can preclude introduction of a significant number of bacteria.

Blood Transfusion in the Young Infant

Whole Blood versus Red Blood Cells

For the most part, neonatal and pediatric medical transfusions should be given as red blood cells. The possible exception is the anemic infant with severe hemorrhagic disease of the newborn, for whom a 15 ml/kg transfusion of whole blood less than five days old will correct the anemia and be sufficient to achieve adequate levels of the vitamin K-dependent coagulation factors.

With the advent of the newborn intensive care unit, the number of small infants requiring transfusions to replace blood drawn for laboratory studies has increased considerably. With this increase has come a debate over the most efficient method to provide repeated small transfusions to sick infants. One method is to find a compatible "walking donor" who is typed, has a negative STS and hepatitis B antigen (HBsAg) screening, and is willing to "donate" small amounts of blood, drawn into a heparinized syringe.[12] Negative factors of this approach include loss of control over: arm preparation by the transfusion service; precise amount of anticoagulant used; crossmatching; maintenance of precise records; and the difficulty of preparing packed cells in a syringe. Furthermore, the neonate is extremely sensitive to the action of heparin and can be dangerously anticoagulated by the heparin in the syringe. Safe and efficient use of a single donation can be achieved by drawing a unit of blood into a quadruple pack.[13] Each satellite can be used more than once within a 24-hour period; thus, an infant can be given multiple transfusions over a three-week period from a single donor. The availability of a 24-hour-a-day microchemistry laboratory can significantly reduce the need for blood transfusion in the Neonatal Intensive Care Unit.

Another approach to the transfusion of the neonate is the use of frozen red blood cells. Such red blood cells, if frozen within five days of collection, are of high quality in that they have excellent posttransfusion viability as well as optimal hemoglobin function, because their levels of ATP and 2,3-DPG are maintained while they are in the frozen state. In addition, because the process of deglycerolization by washing results in removal of supernatant plasma and additives, the problems of citrate

131

overload, transfusion of excessive potassium, or of microaggregates, are largely avoided. In addition, it appears that the risk of transmission of disease, especially hepatitis, is somewhat reduced with transfusion of frozen red blood cells. It also appears likely that the risk of cytomegalovirus disease can be decreased with transfusion of frozen red blood cells.

Choice of Route of Transfusion

The veins used in transfusing older children and adults are frequently inaccessible in young infants, and alternate routes must be selected. The umbilical vessels are most frequently catheterized for intravenous therapy in the neonatal ICU. In addition, scalp veins are used in young infants, as are the veins of the dorsal venous network of the wrist. Finally, the great saphenous vein can be used in older infants and young children.

When a vein is needed for short-term infusion or transfusion, particularly in toddlers, inserting a "butterfly" needle into an external jugular vein can be accomplished easily, and in a child who is not thrashing about, there is little likelihood of perforating the vein if a moderate amount of head and neck movement is allowed.

Transfusion into the tibial marrow cavity, and intraperitoneal transfusion are other possibilities. Each is acceptable if intravenous administration is not possible.

Dosage

Transfusion dosages for infants and young children are best determined from body weight. In general, young infants can tolerate a transfusion volume of 10 to 15ml/kg given in 90 to 150 minutes. In older infants and children, transfusions can be given in amounts up to 20 ml/kg. Unless there is reason to believe that the patient is suffering from cardiopulmonary disease, this amount can be administered in 90 to 150 minutes. Where incipient or actual cardiac decompensation is present, transfusion rates should be limited to no more than 5 ml/kg/hour, and the amount transfused limited to 5 to 10 ml/kg at any one time.

Formulas which recommend different transfusion volumes based on whether the transfusion is to be of packed cells or whole blood are not based on any scientific evidence that an infant or child can tolerate whole blood better than packed cells. Obviously, a transfusion of packed cells will produce almost twice the increment in hemoglobin obtained with whole blood.

Transfusion of one ml of packed cells per kilo will increase the PCV by one; 3 ml/kg of packed cells will raise the hemoglobin by 1 gm/dl. During the neonatal period, these calculations will result in hemoglobin-hematocrit increments that are about 15% lower than the calculation.

132

Age of Blood for Transfusion

When transfusing youngsters with chronic hemolytic anemia, such as thalassemia, it is desirable to achieve the maximum hemoglobin increment with the least iron load. This can best be achieved with blood that has not aged for three weeks. Since many of these patients have severe febrile transfusion reactions, the use of frozen red cells can solve both the problem of "freshness" and reduction of nonerythroid antigenic material.

Since small premature infants may receive relatively large amounts of blood to replace that removed for laboratory study, packed red cells less than five days old are generally recommended. For children receiving blood for surgical or traumatic hemorrhage, or for self-limited hemolysis (eg, G6PD deficiency with acute hemolysis), the age of the blood used is not critical, and there should be no restriction on the use of routine banked blood.

Choice of Blood for Chronic Blood Users

Youngsters entering chronic transfusion programs (as for thalassemia), should be genotyped for the blood group antigens most likely to cause allosensitization. These include the Rh antigens, Fy^a, Kell, and Jk^a. When possible, blood selected for transfusion of these patients should not contain these antigens unless they are present in the patient.

Platelet Transfusion in Infancy

The most common causes of neonatal thrombocytopenia include RDS, sepsis, congenital virus infections, immunothrombocytopenia, and disseminated intravascular coagulation.

Isoimmunization of the mother to a specific platelet group inherited by the infant from its father, or preceding ITP in the mother, are the usual mechanisms for immunothrombocytopenia. The need for platelet transfusion in these infants can generally be determined by evaluating the clinical status of the baby, as well as the platelet count. Where frank hemorrhage is noted and the thrombocytopenia is an isolated finding in the coagulation workup, platelet concentrate is indicated. Washed maternal platelets suspended in AB plasma have been used to treat infants with isoimmune thrombocytopenia. "Fresh" blood is not a useful product, since the number of platelets in whole blood is too small to satisfy the needs of thrombocytopenic patients, unless an exchange transfusion is performed. The routine use of platelet concentrates to treat the thrombocytopenia seen in infants after exchange transfusion would appear to have little merit, in the absence of overt hemorrhage.

133

While the indications for platelet concentrates in pediatric patients are generally the same as those in adults, the infant may present special problems. First, the transfusion of ABO-incompatible plasma which usually presents no problem to the adult patient may produce hemolysis in the small recipient. It is, therefore, wise to transfuse platelets from donors whose plasma is ABO-compatible with the baby. Second, because the volume of platelet concentrates stored at room temperature ranges from 30 ml to 50 ml, it may be difficult to transfuse adequate numbers of platelets to thrombocytopenic infants without producing fluid overload. In such cases, platelet concentrates can be specially prepared for the pediatric patient in a small volume of plasma (15 ml to 20 ml). These platelets should be transfused as soon as possible after preparation. Platelet concentrates can be centrifuged immediately prior to transfusion, permitting removal of 15 ml to 30 ml of supernatant plasma.

Since one platelet concentrate per five kilograms will raise the platelet count by almost 100,000/mm, the problem of "overload" has probably been exaggerated. At maximum PC volume (50 ml), if this formula is used, an infant would receive 11 ml/kg, which can usually be handled without stressing the cardiovascular system. It should be noted that 11 ml/kg of freshly prepared PC also contain therapeutic amounts of all the coagulation factors for a small infant.

Granulocyte Transfusion in Infancy

The usefulness of granulocyte transfusion in nonmalignant neonatal neutropenia has not been evaluated. Indications for granulocyte transfusion in young patients with leukemia, aplastic anemia, or immunosuppressed bone marrow are essentially the same as in adults (Chapter 10). Recently, granulocyte transfusion has been used with apparent success in a non-neutropenic patient with chronic granulomatous disease.[14]

Aside from the greater ease with which substantial increments in white cell count can be achieved with the same pheresis products, there are no known specific differences between granulocyte transfusion in adults and in children.[14]

Coagulation Factor Replacement

Hemorrhagic tendencies are frequent in the neonatal period. All infants have some degree of deficiency of the vitamin K-dependent coagulation factors and this is particularly true in premature infants who have experienced hypoxia.

The observed abnormalities in prothrombin time and partial thromboplastin time appear at birth, become worse at 48 to 72 hours, and then spontaneously remit. If vitamin K is given at birth, these changes are minimized in the healthy full-term infants, but significant depression of Factors II, VII, IX, and X may be seen in sick prematures despite vitamin K administration.

When oozing from the umbilical cord, puncture sites, nose or gastro-intestinal tract is seen, hemorrhagic disease of the newborn has become manifest. When the bleeding occurs in a sick premature infant who has received vitamin K, additional doses are unlikely to be effective and 10 to 12 ml/kg of fresh, fresh frozen, or cryodepleted frozen plasma should be transfused. It is wise to remember that central nervous system bleeding can occur in infants with neonatal hemorrhagic disease, and procrastination in reversing the coagulopathy may result in a brain-damaged baby.

In addition to the temporary deficiency of the vitamin K-dependent factors, any of the hereditary coagulation factor deficiencies may become manifest at birth, since the coagulation factors do not traverse the placenta from mother to infant. Any unusual tendency to bruising, oozing from skin punctures, or mucous membranes in neonates should be evaluated.

Although congenital Factor XIII (FSF) deficiency is a rare disease, it characteristically presents with isolated hemorrhage from the umbilical stump, appearing at 4 to 10 days of age, which is later than the umbilical bleeding due to hemorrhagic disease of the newborn.

Summary

The development of neonatal intensive care units has been accompanied by a significant increase in the number of transfusions given to sick new-borns. At the present time, it appears that providing blood for the neonatal ICU has become the most difficult problem for the hospital transfusion service, replacing the difficulties in providing for cardio-pulmonary surgical needs. This is accentuated by the newness of some of the indications for neonatal transfusion, and by the differences of opinion among neonatologists concerning what constitutes an ideal trans-fusion product for a sick newborn.

The demand for multiple small aliquots of "fresh" blood can create severe logistical problems and has led to seeking new ways to collect and maintain blood for these patients. The daily collection of group O blood in "quad" packs by hospitals and community blood centers has proved to be the most satisfactory technic for meeting these demands, and in general seems preferable to the routine use of frozen red blood cells, or a walking donor pool.

Irradiation of blood being used for intrauterine transfusion has become almost routine, and it seems likely that a similar regimen should apply to any platelet or granulocyte concentrate given to newborn infants.

The survival rate among small and/or very sick neonates has improved dramatically during the past decade. The transfusion has been an important factor in achieving this success.

References

1. Lang DJ, Valerie CF: Hazards of Blood Transfusion. *Adv Pediatr* 24:311, 1977.
2. Oski FA, Naiman JL: *Hematologic Problems in the Newborn,* ed 2. Philadelphia, W. B. Saunders Co., 1972.
3. Burman D, Morris AF: Cord haemoglobin in low birthweight infants. *Arch Dis Child* 49:382, 1974.
4. Bowman JM: Rh Erythroblastosis 1975. *Semin Hematol* 12:189, 1975.
5. Ford JM, Cullen MH, Lucey JJ, et al: Fatal graft-versus-host disease following transfusions of granulocytes from normal donors. *Lancet* 2:1167, 1976.
6. Button LN, DeWolf W, Jacobson M, et al: Irradiation of Blood Components, abstracted. Proceedings of the 30th Annual Meeting of the American Association of Blood Banks, 1977, p 16.
7. Telischi M, Krmpotic E, Moss G: Viable lymphocytes in frozen washed blood. *Transfusion* 15:481, 1975.
8. Maisels MJ: Bilirubin: On understanding and influencing its metabolism in the newborn infant. *Pediatr Clin North Am* 19:447, 1972.
9. Milner RDG: Neonatal metabolism and endocrinology studied by exchange transfusion. *Clin Endocrinol Metabol* 5:221, 1976.
10. Hathaway WE: The bleeding newborn. *Semin Hematol* 12:175, 1975.
11. Delivoria-Papadopoulos M, Miller LD, Forster RD, et al: The role of exchange transfusion in the management to low-birthweight infants with and without severe respiratory disease syndrome. *J Pediatr* 89:273, 1976.
12. Hattersley PG, Goetzman BW, Gross S, et al: A walking blood donor program for seriously ill premature infants. *Transfusion* 16:366, 1976.
13. Oberman, HA: Replacement transfusion in the newborn infant: A Commentary. *J Pediatr* 86:586, 1975.
14. Maybee DA, Millan AP, Ruymann FB: Granulocyte transfusion therapy in children. *South Med J,* 70:3, 1977.
15. Bharucha C, Cherian M, Bauman JH: Congenital deficiency of Factor VIII in an Indian kindred. *Scand J Haematol,* 7:325, 1970.

Chapter 14

ADVERSE REACTIONS TO BLOOD TRANSFUSION

Dennis Goldfinger, MD

Introduction

THE TRANSFUSION of blood components carries with it many
potential risks. Patients may experience adverse reactions to both
the cellular and noncellular constituents of blood; many such reactions
are immunologically mediated. A variety of diseases may be transmitted
from the donor to the recipient. Infection also may be transmitted to
the recipient by contamination of the blood during collection or storage.
The anticoagulants and preservatives, as well as the accumulated products
of cellular metabolism and breakdown, may cause undesired effects.
Whenever the decision is made to transfuse a blood component, the
relative hazards of the transfusion should be balanced against the possible
benefits to the recipient. Only when the patient is clearly in need of transfusion, and the potential value outweighs the risks, should the component
be transfused.

Signs and Symptoms of Transfusion Reactions

Signs and symptoms of adverse reactions to blood transfusion may
include fever, shaking chills, hives, dyspnea, pain in the back, chest or
elsewhere, hypertension, hypotension or shock. If a transfusion reaction
is suspected, it is most important that the transfusion be stopped immediately in order to minimize the amount of blood infused into the patient.
The intravenous line should be kept open with saline solution while the
reaction is being evaluated.

Clinical and Laboratory Evaluation

The transfusion reaction workup is designed primarily to detect whether
a hemolytic reaction has occurred. The evaluation of transfusion reactions
should proceed rapidly, since early diagnosis of acute hemolytic reactions
can allow the physician to institute preventive therapy to avert complications. Furthermore, rapid diagnosis of nonhemolytic, clinically insignificant reactions can avoid unnecessary delays in providing additional blood
for transfusion to the patient. For this reason, the protocol for clinical

137

and laboratory evaluation of suspected transfusion reactions can be divided into two parts. In most cases, an initial, rapid, and rather simple evaluation can determine if a hemolytic transfusion reaction has occurred. A more elaborate evaluation can be performed only in those cases where, on the basis of the initial evaluation, it is suspected that the patient may have suffered a clinically significant reaction. Generally, only the initial, abbreviated portion of the workup needs to be done, since the likelihood of a potentially dangerous reaction is ruled out by the preliminary evaluation. This approach saves time for the technologist and, more importantly, allows the patient to receive additional transfusions, if needed, without dangerous delays.

The initial evaluation of suspected transfusion reactions should include the following:

1. To prevent further infusion of possibly incompatible blood, discontinue the transfusion. The intravenous line may be kept open with a saline drip.
2. Clinical evaluation of the patient should be made by a physician or nurse. Patients having severe and dangerous reactions usually will have prominent signs and symptoms.
3. A clerical check should be performed at the patient's bedside. It may become apparent immediately that the patient is receiving the wrong unit of blood.
4. A blood sample should be drawn carefully (to prevent hemolysis) and sent to the blood bank with the empty or partially empty bag of blood.
5. A clerical check should be performed in the blood bank to determine if a laboratory error has been made, resulting in transfusion of the wrong unit of blood to the patient.
6. The posttransfusion blood sample should be centrifuged, and the plasma examined for the presence of free hemoglobin. Visual examination will detect levels of hemoglobinemia of 25-50 mg/dl, as a distinctly red color. This level will be produced by intravascular lysis of only 5 ml to 10 ml of red blood cells in an adult. Chemical determinations of plasma-free hemoglobin usually should not be performed, since the results are often misleading (improper specimen collection or handling can produce false elevations above the normal range).
7. The posttransfusion plasma should be examined visually for icterus. Bilirubin levels will be elevated within a few hours, following a significant episode of hemolysis.
8. The ABO group of the posttransfusion blood sample and the unit

138

of blood implicated in the reaction should be determined. The majority of serious acute hemolytic transfusion reactions are the result of ABO incompatible transfusion.

9. A direct antiglobulin (Coombs) test should be performed on the postreaction blood specimen.

Tests on the pretransfusion blood sample, such as ABO grouping, antibody screening and recrossmatching probably need not be performed unless discrepancies are found in the posttransfusion sample or unit of transfused blood. Also, antibody screening and crossmatching, utilizing the posttransfusion blood sample, probably need not be performed if the above evaluation shows no evidence of an acute hemolytic transfusion reaction.

If these preliminary studies are unremarkable, it is probable that no other investigations need be carried out. However, if results are found suggesting that a hemolytic or other serious transfusion reaction has occurred, additional studies might be indicated. These may include ABO grouping of the pretransfusion blood sample, antibody screening and crossmatching with pre- and posttransfusion blood samples, including minor crossmatching, direct antiglobulin testing of the prereaction blood specimen, examination of the patient's urine for free hemoglobin, gram stain and culture of the transfused unit of blood, and other studies, as deemed necessary.

Acute Hemolytic Transfusion Reactions

The acute hemolytic transfusion reaction is among the complications most feared in blood transfusion therapy. The serious sequelae which may follow such reactions are acute renal failure, due to acute tubular necrosis; and a hemorrhagic diathesis, which may be of life-threatening proportions. The most serious hemolytic transfusion reactions usually are due to ABO incompatibility; however, other blood group incompatibility may result in equally severe reactions. The most common cause for ABO-incompatible transfusion is clerical error (ie, transfusing the wrong unit of blood to the patient); therefore, meticulous care in the steps leading to transfusion, including specimen collection, is by far the best single means of minimizing the risk of an acute hemolytic reaction. If it is suspected that an acute hemolytic transfusion reaction has occurred, the most important consideration in treatment is to minimize the dose of incompatible blood transfused; therefore, the blood transfusion should be stopped immediately.

Previously, it had been hypothesized that the acute renal failure following incompatible transfusion resulted either from obstruction of the renal

139

tubules by hemoglobin casts, or from a direct toxic effect of hemoglobin on the tubular epithelium. It is now clear, however, that neither of these factors is important. Instead, the renal failure appears to result from ischemic damage to the tubules which, in turn, is caused by disseminated intravascular coagulation and a series of vasomotor alterations which decrease renal cortical blood flow. These circulatory changes probably are brought about by the release of vasoactive compounds which produce systemic hypotension and specific alterations in the blood flow to the kidneys. These are identical to the hemodynamic aberrations seen in shock from any other causes (eg, sepsis, hemorrhage). The activation of the coagulation system and the release of vasoactive compounds are triggered by the antigen-antibody reaction, often with participation of the complement system.[1,2]

Although diuretics (especially mannitol), by their ability to increase urine flow and "flush out" the kidney, have been advocated as "preventive" treatment to avert renal shutdown following acute hemolytic transfusion reactions, such therapy has little rationale in light of current knowledge of the pathogenetic mechanisms involved. Instead, vigorous treatment of hypotension, similar to that used in more common forms of shock, should be the most important consideration. Intravenous infusion of fluids combined with administration of vasoactive drugs, such as dopamine, seems to be the soundest approach to therapy. While certain diuretics have been thought to increase renal cortical perfusion, in addition to augmenting urine flow, the evidence for such an effect is controversial. At any rate, increased renal cortical blood flow has been demonstrated more convincingly for furosemide than for mannitol.[2]

In order to avert the complication of disseminated intravascular coagulation following incompatible transfusion, heparin can be administered "prophylactically" in such cases.[1,2] It is likely that anticoagulant therapy is beneficial only if given very early, before significant intravascular coagulation has commenced.[3] Since use of heparin is contraindicated in many patients who may receive incompatible blood (ie, in postoperative bleeding, or trauma), each case must be individualized, with the potential benefits weighed against the possible risks.

When an acute hemolytic transfusion reaction is suspected, an attempt should be made, as rapidly as possible, to determine the severity of the reaction. The following factors should receive primary consideration:

1. Severe reactions are likely to be accompanied by prominent signs and symptoms. The development of hypotension and shock is an ominous sign.
2. The volume of incompatible red blood cells infused is of critical

140

importance—severe sequelae rarely follow the transfusion of less than one-half to one unit (100 ml to 250 ml) of packed red blood cells (200 ml to 500 ml of whole blood).

3. A posttransfusion blood sample usually will show visible hemoglobinemia, if a significant reaction has occurred.

When a serious acute hemolytic transfusion reaction has been confirmed, the following steps may be used in treatment:

1. Avoid further transfusion of incompatible red blood cells.
2. Treat hypovolemia and hypotension by intravenous infusion of fluids (colloids or crystalloids).
3. Consider the administration of dopamine to combat systemic hypotension and improve renal cortical blood flow.
4. Consider the administration of diuretics (furosemide or mannitol) to augment renal blood flow.
5. Consider the "prophylactic" administration of heparin to prevent disseminated intravascular coagulation. If significant intravascular clotting has begun already, anticoagulation may be of no benefit. Heparin therapy needs to be continued only so long as the stimulus for coagulation is likely to be present (probably not more than 6 to 12 hours).
6. If renal shutdown occurs, and cannot be reversed, standard therapy for acute tubular necrosis, including fluid restriction, should be instituted.

Alloimmunization

Immunization to erythrocyte alloantigens is an unavoidable risk of red blood cell transfusion. Patients may become sensitized and produce antibodies to any red blood cell antigens which they lack, and which are present on the transfused cells. Following such antibody formation, future transfusion is made more difficult since it will become necessary to select units of blood lacking the corresponding antigen. If blood containing the specific antigen is transferred, a serious hemolytic transfusion reaction might result. In addition, these antibodies may produce hemolytic disease of the newborn in future pregnancies.

Most antibodies of clinical significance are of the IgG class of immunoglobulins. Antibodies may be formed to antigens of the Rh, Kell, Duffy, Kidd, or other blood group systems. The risk of sensitization has been found to be approximately 1% for each unit of blood transfused[4]; therefore, a patient receiving 20 units of blood has about a 20% chance of forming a red blood cell antibody.

141

Since the reactivity of unexpected red blood cell antibodies can diminish with time, their presence may be missed at the time of future transfusion. This may result in the transfusion of incompatible blood and a delayed or acute hemolytic transfusion reaction. To protect sensitized patients from the hazard of an incompatible transfusion, these patients should be informed that they possess a red blood cell antibody. Some investigators have found it useful to give such patients a wallet card indicating the specificity of the antibody, so that this information can be conveyed to physicians who may be transfusing such patients in the future.[5]

Delayed Hemolytic Transfusion Reactions

Delayed hemolytic transfusion reactions may occur in one of two ways. The first, and milder, form occurs in conjunction with primary alloimmunization. After red blood cell transfusion, exposure of the recipient to foreign antigens may result in sensitization and antibody production. Characteristically, there is a lag period of at least ten days to two weeks (often much longer) before antibody production begins. As antibody concentration rises, a reaction may occur with circulating transfused red blood cells. This may result in accelerated destruction of these transfused cells, the rate of hemolysis being dependent mainly on the quantity of antibody produced. However, destruction is rarely very rapid, because the rate of antibody production is usually not great. In most cases, the accelerated red blood cell destruction goes unnoticed. Laboratory studies, if properly timed, may show a decrease in hemoglobin concentration, mild hyperbilirubinemia, a positive direct antiglobulin (Coombs) test, and the appearance of red blood cell alloantibodies in the serum.

The second form of delayed hemolytic transfusion reaction results from a secondary or anamnestic response to a foreign antigen on transfused red blood cells.[5,6] Following primary sensitization to a red blood cell antigen, reexposure to that same antigen, months or years later, may result in a booster response in antibody synthesis. The characteristics of this anamnestic response are rapid antibody production with a short lag period (one to five days), and relatively greater amounts of antibody produced as compared to primary immunization. Since significant quantities of antibody will be produced while large numbers of incompatible red blood cells are still circulating, a marked degree of red blood cell destruction may occur. This may result in a rapid fall in hemoglobin concentration, associated with hyperbilirubinemia (and, at times, clinical jaundice). Hemolysis usually takes place extravascularly (in macrophages), but on rare occasion, intravascular lysis may occur, with resultant hemoglobinuria.[7] A positive direct antiglobulin test will

142

be found, unless all of the incompatible red blood cells have been destroyed by the time the test is performed. A rising concentration of antibody will be detected in the patient's serum in the days to follow; this may be diagnostically helpful in deciding whether a delayed hemolytic transfusion reaction has occurred.

Delayed hemolytic transfusion reactions rarely result in dangerous sequelae, although there have been a few reports of acute renal failure following such reactions.[5,6,8] Disseminated intravascular coagulation and shock, common complications of acute hemolytic transfusion reactions, rarely, if ever, occur following delayed hemolytic transfusion reactions. Undoubtedly, the reaction proceeds too slowly under these circumstances to produce significant activation of the coagulation system or to trigger the release of large quantities of vasoactive compounds. A single report of disseminated intravascular coagulation due to a delayed hemolytic transfusion reaction[6] provides too few details to be evaluated adequately.

The greatest potential danger of delayed hemolytic transfusion reactions lies in predisposing the patient to a subsequent acute hemolytic transfusion reaction. It may not be realized, as hemoglobin concentration falls, that the etiology of the anemia is immunologically mediated hemolysis. Other causes (eg, occult bleeding) are suspected instead, and additional transfusions may be prescribed. If further transfusions are given with incompatible red blood cells, an acute hemolytic transfusion reaction could ensue, since the patient now has a higher concentration of red blood cell antibodies in the plasma.[5] The practice of obtaining repeated serum samples for crossmatching, whenever patients are receiving repeated transfusions, can prevent such acute hemolytic reactions by detecting newly developing antibodies, thereby averting the transfusion of additional incompatible blood.[9]

Febrile, Nonhemolytic Transfusion Reactions

Fever, often associated with chills, occurring during or shortly after transfusion, is the most common form of transfusion reaction. Such reactions frequently are caused by antibodies to white blood cells, and are encountered most often in multitransfused or multiparous patients.[10,11] While these reactions usually are not dangerous in themselves, they are certainly a great discomfort to the recipients of blood transfusion. In addition, they can result in serious delays in providing additional blood for transfusion, since they must be differentiated from reactions due to transfusion of contaminated blood and from acute hemolytic transfusion reactions. Therefore, if the recipient of a blood transfusion should develop chills or fever, the transfusion should be stopped immediately and the reaction promptly investigated to rule out the possibility that a hemolytic reaction has occurred. If appropriate studies reveal that a febrile non-hemolytic transfusion reaction has occurred, then, leukocyte-poor red blood cells generally will prevent further reactions. Antihistamines (eg, Benadryl) probably have no value in the prevention or treatment of these reactions. Leukocyte-poor red blood cells can be supplied either as buffy coat-poor, saline-washed, or frozen red blood cells.

Urticarial Transfusion Reactions

Urticarial reactions are the second most frequently encountered reactions to blood transfusion. The cause for such reactions remains unknown, but most investigators feel that the reactions are related to allergy to a soluble product contained in the donor plasma. Transfusion reactions consisting solely of urticaria are not dangerous, and need not be investigated as possible hemolytic transfusion reactions; however, if urticaria is associated with fever and/or chills, then the possibility of a hemolytic reaction must be considered and appropriate investigative measures undertaken. Generally, patients who have had urticarial transfusion reactions should be treated with an antihistamine (eg, Benadryl, 50 mg intramuscularly) prior to transfusion, or should receive washed or frozen red blood cells, which are largely devoid of plasma.[12]

Circulatory Overload

Volume overload, due to transfusion of too much blood too quickly, is probably a very frequent complication of blood transfusion therapy, although such reactions often are not diagnosed, and, frequently, are not reported to the transfusion service. Symptoms may include acute dyspnea, a feeling of tightness in the chest, and headache. The patient's blood pressure may become elevated, and there may be physical and radiographic evidence of frank pulmonary edema. These reactions occur most frequently in elderly patients with poor cardiac reserve, although they may occur in young patients with no history of heart disease. Heart failure, once it occurs, can be irreversible and fatal.

Such reactions are completely preventable in most instances, simply by avoiding the transfusion of large volumes of whole blood or plasma to normovolemic patients. While bleeding or hypovolemic patients may receive whole blood, nonbleeding anemic patients should receive only packed, washed or frozen red blood cells. Washed or frozen red blood cells contain no plasma, thereby decreasing the oncotic load to the patient.[12] Transfusions should be given slowly (2 to 3 hours per unit), and, except in unusual circumstances, not more than two units of blood (or a

144

maximum of three) should be transfused per day to stable, nonbleeding patients—even those with severe anemia. There is no need for rapid transfusion of excessive quantities of blood no matter how anemic the patient.

Infectious Complications of Transfusion

Posttransfusion Hepatitis

Posttransfusion hepatitis remains the most frequent serious complication of blood transfusion. It is difficult to estimate the magnitude of the problem since the majority of cases are anicteric and subclinical. However, recent reports from a number of institutions have demonstrated an alarmingly high rate of hepatitis in carefully followed groups of transfusion recipients. Even more disturbing is the frequent occurrence of chronic active hepatitis, following anicteric, subclinical, posttransfusion hepatitis.[13]

With the institution of universal testing for hepatitis B surface antigen (HBsAg) in this country, it is clear that the majority of posttransfusion hepatitis seen today is not due to the hepatitis B virus. Also, because of the availability of tests to detect the hepatitis A virus it is evident that very little, if any, posttransfusion hepatitis is due to that virus. Evidently, there are other viruses capable of causing posttransfusion hepatitis, and these viruses are considered responsible for most of the current cases of this disease (so-called "non-A, non-B hepatitis").[13,14]

Blood products capable of causing posttransfusion hepatitis include whole blood, all red blood cell-containing products, fresh frozen plasma, stored plasma, fibrinogen, cryoprecipitated antihemophilic factor, Factor VIII concentrate, Factor IX (prothrombin complex) concentrate, platelet concentrate, and granulocyte concentrate. The high incidence of hepatitis following transfusion of fibrinogen is the reason this product is no longer on the market in this country. Immune serum globulin (ISG), manufactured in this country, has never been implicated as a cause of hepatitis and does not contain measurable HBsAg.[15] Although albumin and plasma protein fraction contain HBsAg,[16] they are safe; all albumin for transfusion is heated to 60 C for ten hours, thereby killing the hepatitis virus. While frozen red blood cells are capable of transmitting hepatitis,[17] evidence suggests that the risk is reduced following frozen red blood cell transfusion, as compared to transfusion of other red blood cell products.[18] This decreased risk probably results from removal of hepatitis virus during the extensive washing procedure involved in deglycerolization of frozen red blood cells.[19] Blood products manufactured from pools of

145

The risk of transfusion-transmitted syphilis is considered to be so small that routine serologic testing of donor units is no longer recommended as a worthwhile preventive measure.

Transmission of toxoplasmosis has been reported in patients receiving transfusions of granulocyte concentrates collected from donors with chronic granulocytic leukemia. The patients who acquired the disease through transfusion had been immunosuppressed, which increased their susceptibility to developing such infection. Since the toxoplasma organisms are carried in peripheral blood leukocytes, only blood products containing white blood cells are capable of transmitting this disease. It is not known whether normal donors are likely to have parasitemia, and transmit toxoplasmosis, since, in the reported cases, the granulocyte donors had diseases which may have made them susceptible to ongoing parasitemia by these organisms.[30]

Transfusion of Contaminated Blood

Current methods of collecting, processing, and storing blood components have made administration of massively contaminated blood a very rare complication of transfusion therapy. In the event of transfusion with heavily contaminated blood, the patient immediately will develop severe septic shock, a reaction that is frequently fatal. If septic shock is suspected, rapid measures should be instituted to save the patient, including immediate cessation of blood transfusion and supportive measures to combat infection and shock.

Transfusion of blood components contaminated by very small numbers of viable bacteria does not result in a symptomatic reaction in the majority of patients, but may cause serious reactions in immunosuppressed patients.[31,32] Such patients may be exquisitely sensitive to even very small numbers of viable bacteria. Since this form of reaction usually does not present with acute symptomatology, but rather results in the development of sepsis within hours or days following transfusion of the contaminated blood product, the cause for such sepsis can only be suspected, and may be confirmed only by culture of the involved blood products, if available. The incidence of this form of reaction is unknown, but its existence provides another reason for minimizing the frequency of blood transfusion, whenever possible.

Anaphylactic Transfusion Reactions

Patients who have a total deficiency of IgA proteins may form antibodies to the IgA contained in transfused plasma. Once sensitized, reexposure to IgA via blood transfusion may provoke an acute anaphylactic reaction, consisting of flushing, dyspnea, wheezing, severe hypotension, and shock.[33-35] These reactions may be life-threatening, and one fatal reaction has been reported.[33] Patients known to possess anti-IgA antibodies can safely receive only IgA-deficient blood products. These include frozen or saline washed red blood cells, where the IgA proteins have been washed from the red blood cells, or blood collected from IgA-deficient donors.

Patients who are not totally IgA deficient, but lack one of the IgA subclasses, can form anti-IgA antibodies of limited specificity, and have reactions to the IgA subclass which they lack. Such reactions usually are milder in nature.[36] Patients who have had reactions to IgA, and who require plasma-containing blood components (eg, fresh frozen plasma, platelets, immune serum globulin) must receive such components collected from IgA-deficient donors. Registries of such donors are maintained by the Irwin Blood Bank in San Francisco and the American Red Cross.

Graft-Versus-Host Disease

Engraftment and multiplication of donor blood cells may occur following transfusion to immunodeficient patients. Cells of the erythrocytic, granulocytic, or lymphocytic series may engraft and replicate, but such grafts often persist only transiently.[37,38] When immunocompetent lymphocytes become engrafted and cannot be rejected by the immunodeficient host, the engrafted cells may react against the foreign tissues of the transfusion recipient, and graft-versus-host disease (GVH) may develop.

The syndrome of GVH may include fever, skin rash, hepatitis, severe diarrhea, bone marrow suppression, and infection. This complication of blood transfusion may be fatal. GVH can be prevented by irradiating all lymphocyte-containing blood components prior to transfusion (whole blood, packed red blood cells, platelet concentrates and granulocyte concentrates). The administration of 1500-3000 rads will render lymphocytes incapable of replication and division, thereby preventing their engraftment and multiplication in the transfusion recipient.

Until recently, reports of fatal GVH involved only the most highly immunodeficient patients (children with severe combined immunodeficiency, bone marrow transplant recipients, and fetuses receiving intrauterine transfusion).[39,40] Current reports, however, present evidence of GVH in less highly immunosuppressed patients (eg, children receiving high dose chemotherapy for neuroblastoma).[41] If these less highly immunosuppressed patients may acquire GVH from transfusion, irradiation of blood products may be recommended as a precaution for increased numbers of patients in the near future.

149

Noncardiogenic Pulmonary Edema

The development of severe respiratory distress, unassociated with circulatory overload, has been reported as a rare complication of transfusion therapy. In such cases, the patient develops typical signs and symptoms of acute pulmonary edema during or shortly after transfusion, but without evidence of cardiac failure. Chest x-rays demonstrate bilateral pulmonary infiltrates, consistent with pulmonary edema, but without other evidence of left heart failure.[42,43] These reactions may be extremely severe, taking several days for the patient to recover totally from the episode; fatal episodes of this reaction have been reported.[44] The etiology of the pulmonary edema is not known, but the most prevalent hypothesis is that the reaction is due to leukocyte antibodies—either antibodies possessed by the recipient and directed against transfused leukocytes; or antibodies contained in donor plasma, which react with the recipient's own white blood cells. While the optimal approach to therapy is not known, treatment probably should be similar to that used for pulmonary edema resulting from heart failure. Patients who have suffered from this type of transfusion reaction probably should receive leukocyte-poor blood products for future transfusion.

Hemosiderosis

Hemosiderosis is a potential risk for patients who will receive many units of blood over a considerable period of time. This complication is controlled most effectively by minimizing the number of transfusions given to chronically anemic patients. Reduction of accumulated iron stores with iron chelating agents, eg, desferrioxamine, may be of value, but treatment remains controversial.

Air Embolism

The use of modern transfusion equipment, including plastic blood bags, minimizes the risk of air embolism in transfusion recipients. Currently, the only significant risk of air embolism occurs when blood is administered under pressure infusion. The signs and symptoms of air embolism include acute shortness of breath, chest pain, syncope and shock. Of course, patients receiving blood under pressure infusion are likely to be in severe distress and may not exhibit the usual symptoms of this complication; sudden, unexpected respiratory distress and hypotension may be the only signs encountered. Treatment of air embolism consists of immediate prevention of additional air entering the circulation and placement of the patient on the left side, with feet elevated. This position tends to localize the air to the apex of the right ventricle, thereby keeping it out of the pulmonary outflow tract. The patient should be given 100% oxygen to breathe.

References

1. Goldfinger D: Complications of hemolytic transfusion reactions: Pathogenesis and therapy, in Dawson RB (ed); *New Approaches to Transfusion Reactions*. Washington, DC, American Association of Blood Banks, 1974.
2. Goldfinger D: Acute hemolytic transfusion reactions—A fresh look at pathogenesis and considerations regarding therapy. *Transfusion* 17:85-98, 1977.
3. Rock RC, Bove JR, Nemerson Y: Heparin treatment of intravascular coagulation accompanying hemolytic transfusion reactions. *Transfusion* 9:57-61, 1969.
4. Lostumbo MM, Holland PV, Schmidt PJ: Isoimmunization after multiple transfusions. *N Engl J Med* 275:141-144, 1966.
5. Solanki D, McCurdy PR: Delayed hemolytic transfusion reactions. An often-missed entity. *JAMA* 239:729-731, 1978.
6. Pineda AA, Taswell HF, Brzica SM Jr: Delayed hemolytic transfusion reaction. An immunologic hazard of blood transfusion. *Transfusion* 18:1-7, 1978.
7. Pickles MM, Jones MH, Egan J, et al: Delayed hemolytic transfusion reactions due to anti-C. *Vox Sang* 35:32-35, 1978.
8. Holland PV, Wallerstein RO: Delayed hemolytic transfusion reaction with acute renal failure. *JAMA* 204:1007-1008, 1968.
9. Oberman HA (ed): *Standards for Blood Banks and Transfusion Services,* ed 9. Washington, DC, American Association of Blood Banks, 1978.
10. Brittingham TE, Chaplin H Jr: Febrile transfusion reactions caused by sensitivity to donor leukocytes and platelets. *JAMA* 165:819-825, 1957.
11. Perkins, HA, Payne R, Ferguson J, et al: Nonhemolytic febrile transfusion reactions. Quantitative effects of blood components with emphasis on isoantigenic incompatibility of leukocytes. *Vox Sang* 11:578-600, 1966.
12. Goldfinger D, Lowe C: Prevention of adverse reactions to blood transfusion by the administration of saline washed red blood cells. *Transfusion,* in press.
13. Alter HJ, Purcell RH, Feinstone SM, et al: Non-A/non-B hepatitis: A review and interim report of an ongoing prospective study, in

Vyas GN, Cohen SN, Schmid R (eds): *Viral Hepatitis.* Philadelphia, The Franklin Institute Press, 1978, pp 359-369.

14. Feinstone SM, Kapikian AZ, Purcell RH, et al: Transfusion-associated hepatitis not due to viral hepatitis type A or B. *N Engl J Med* 292:767-770, 1975.
15. Holland PV, Alter HJ, Purcell RH, et al: Hepatitis B antigen (HBsAg) and antibody (anti-HBsAg) in cold ethanol fractions of human plasma. *Transfusion* 12:363-370, 1972.
16. Hoofnagle JH, Barker LF, Thiel J, et al: Hepatitis B virus and hepatitis B surface antigen in human albumin products. *Transfusion* 16:141-147, 1976.
17. Alter HJ, Tabor E, Meryman HT, et al: Transmission of hepatitis B virus infection by transfusion of frozen-deglycerolized red blood cells. *N Engl J Med* 298:637-642, 1978.
18. Tullis JL, Hinman J, Sproul MT, et al: Incidence of posttransfusion hepatitis in previously frozen blood. *JAMA* 214:719-723, 1970.
19. Contreras TJ, Valeri CR: Removal of HBsAg from blood in vitro. I. Effects of washing alone, glycerol addition and removal, and glycerolization, freezing, and washing. *Transfusion* 16:594-609, 1976.
20. Walsh JH, Purcell RH, Morrow AG, et al: Posttransfusion hepatitis after open-heart operations. *JAMA* 211:261-265, 1970.
21. Holland PV, Rubinson RM, Morrow AG, et al: Gamma globulin in the prophylaxis of posttransfusion hepatitis. *JAMA* 196:471-474, 1966.
22. Katz R, Rodriguez J, Ward R: Posttransfusion hepatitis—effect of modified gamma globulin added to blood in vitro. *N Engl J Med* 285:925-932, 1971.
23. Grady GF, Rodman M, Larsen LH: Hepatitis B antibody in conventional gamma globulin. *J Infect Dis* 132:474-477, 1975.
24. Knodell RG, Conrad ME, Ginsberg AL, et al: Efficacy of prophylactic gamma globulin in preventing non-A, non-B posttransfusion hepatitis. *Lancet* 1.557-567, 1976.
25. Seeff LB, Zimmerman HJ, Wright EC, et al: A randomized, double blind controlled trial of the efficacy of immune serum globulin for the prevention of posttransfusion hepatitis. *Gastroenterology* 72:111-121, 1977.
26. Alter HJ, Barker LF, Holland PV: Hepatitis B immune globulin: Evaluation of clinical trials and rationale for usage. *N Engl J Med* 293:1093-1094, 1975.
27. Weller TH: The cytomegaloviruses: Ubiquitous agents with protean clinical manifestations. *N Engl J Med* 285:203-214, 1971.

28. Foster KM, Jack I: A prospective study of the role of cytomegalovirus in post-transfusion mononucleosis. *N Engl J Med* 280:1311-1316, 1969.

29. Chambers RW, Foley HT, Schmidt PJ: Transmission of syphilis by fresh blood components. *Transfusion* 9:32-34, 1969.

30. Siegel SE, Lunde MN, Gelderman AH: Transmission of toxoplasmosis by leukocyte transfusion. *Blood* 37:388-394, 1971.

31. Buchholz DH, Young VM, Friedman NR, et al: Bacterial proliferation in platelet products stored at room temperature. *N Engl J Med* 285:429-433, 1971.

32. Rhame FS, Root PK, MacLowery JD, et al: An epidemic of septicemia due to Salmonella cholerae—suis var Kunzendorf. Eleventh Inter-Science Conference on Antimicrobial Agents and Chemotherapy, Atlantic City, NJ, 1971.

33. Pineda AA, Taswell HF: Transfusion reactions associated with anti-IgA antibodies: Report of four cases and review of the literature. *Transfusion* 15:10-15, 1975.

34. Schmidt AP, Taswell HF, Gleich GJ: Anaphylactic transfusion reactions associated with anti-IgA antibody. *N Engl J Med* 280:188-193, 1969.

35. Vyas GN, Perkins HA, Fudenberg HH: Anaphylactoid transfusion reactions associated with anti-IgA. *Lancet* 2:312-315, 1968.

36. Vyas GN: Immunological reactions caused by plasma. International Society of Hematology-International Society of Blood Transfusion, Joint Congress, 1978.

37. Bronson WR, McGinniss MH, Morse EE: Hematopoietic graft detected by a change in ABO group. *Blood* 23:239-249, 1964.

38. Schmidt PJ, Yokoyama M, McGinniss MH, et al: Erythroid homograft following leukocyte transfusion in a patient with acute leukemia. II. Serologic and immunochemical studies. *Blood* 26:597-609, 1965.

39. Parkman R, Mosier D, Umansky I, et al: Graft-versus-host disease after intrauterine and exchange transfusions for hemolytic disease of the newborn. *N Engl J Med* 290:359-363, 1974.

40. Naiman JL, Punnett HH, Lischner HW, et al: Possible graft—versus—host reaction after intrauterine transfusion for Rh erythroblastosis fetalis. *N Engl J Med* 281:697-701, 1969.

41. Helson L: Graft versus host disease (GVH) from unirradiated red blood cell and platelet transfusions. International Society of Hematology—International Society of Blood Transfusion, Joint Congress, 1978.

42. Ward HN: Pulmonary infiltrates associated with leukoagglutinin transfusion reactions. *Ann Intern Med* 73:689-694, 1970.

43. Thompson JS, Severson CD, Parmley MJ, et al: Pulmonary "hyper-sensitivity" reactions induced by transfusion of non-HL-A leukoag-glutinins. *N Engl J Med* 284:1120-1125, 1971.
44. Wolf CFW, Canale VC: Fatal pulmonary hypersensitivity reaction to HL-A incompatible blood transfusion: Report of a case and review of the literature. *Transfusion* 16:135-140, 1976.

Chapter 15

THERAPEUTIC PHLEBOTOMY OR REMOVAL OF SELECTED BLOOD COMPONENTS (LEUKAPHERESIS, PLATELETPHERESIS, OR EXCHANGE PLASMAPHERESIS)

Lilian M. Reich, MD

Introduction

THERAPEUTIC REMOVAL of whole blood or its components can usually be accomplished utilizing personnel and equipment from the blood bank or transfusion service. Requests for such procedures require consultation between the medical director of the transfusion service and the physician attending the patient so that there can be agreement on the following points:

1. Valid clinical indication for the procedure.
2. Choice of most appropriate technic(s), where alternatives are available.
3. Facilities and staffing necessary to insure maximum patient safety during the procedure.
4. Parameters to be monitored concerning efficacy of the procedure or possible adverse effects.

Informed consent must be obtained from the patient for each procedure utilized. Usual aseptic donor collection methods should be employed because, under certain circumstances, components removed from the patient may later be issued for autologous or homologous transfusion.

Methods

Manual

Therapeutic phlebotomy can be accomplished manually using appropriate collection sets. Return of the autologous component not to be removed carries the risk of misidentification.

Automated

Therapeutic removal of a selected blood component (leukapheresis, plateletpheresis, or plasmapheresis) is only practical using automated centrifugal blood cell processors. These instruments incur little chance of contamination and no risk of misidentifying the autologous component to be returned. Either one or two venipunctures are employed and heparinization is sometimes necessary.

Continuous flow and intermittent flow centrifugal devices are available. The former have the advantage of a smaller fixed volume ex vivo, and because cell separation is continuous, there is greater cell removal per unit time. In the intermittent flow instrument, because the volume ex vivo is inversely proportional to hematocrit, the therapeutic maneuver may require priming the instrument with compatible red blood cells to prevent hypovolemia during the procedure.

Indications for Therapeutic Phlebotomy

Polycythemia

Removal of whole blood is a frequent modality of therapy in polycythemia vera[1] and is employed under certain circumstances in other polycythemias.[2] It is the treatment of choice when red cell proliferation is the major problem. It is occasionally employed in acute cardiac failure for emergency reduction of circulatory volume.[3]

The rationale for phlebotomy in polycythemias is reduction of whole blood viscosity, which is a function of the hematocrit. In established polycythemia vera, phlebotomy should be considered whenever the patient's hematocrit exceeds 50%. Volume and frequency of venisection require consideration of the patient's blood volume and overall clinical status. Most adults can be brought under control by removing one unit of whole blood one to three times weekly, and then maintaining the patient with periodic phlebotomy of one to three units as the hematocrit rises above 50%. Serial determinations of hemoglobin, hematocrit, and mean corpuscular volume, plus white cell and platelet counts will measure the effectiveness of therapy and warn against a hazardous rise in white cell or platelets, or excessive hypochromia and microcytosis.

In other polycythemias, hyperviscosity may require phlebotomy to maintain an optimal hematocrit. Compensatory polycythemias, in particular, demand highly individualized management, often including a cautious empirical therapeutic trial. Therapeutic phlebotomy is contraindicated in relative or so-called "stress" polycythemia because the hematocrit elevation is a reflection of low plasmacrit.

Hemochromatosis

Therapeutic phlebotomy plays a major role in the management of parenchymal iron overload in conditions other than the iron-loading anemias. These include idiopathic hemochromatosis,[4] most cases of porphyria cutanea tarda,[5] and some cases of transfusion hemosiderosis.[6]

Each unit of blood contains approximately 220 mg of elemental iron. Since repeated phlebotomy induces more rapid red cell proliferation, tissue iron is mobilized for red cell incorporation and, in time, parenchymal iron overload is reduced.

Patients with idiopathic hemochromatosis face a lifelong schedule of venisection therapy. It is the best available technic to expeditiously remove large iron deposits (which may exceed 30 gm). Most patients will tolerate removal of one unit one to two times weekly until controlled. A less intensive maintenance phlebotomy schedule can then be instituted. Removal of three to six units yearly is the usual range for maintenance. Similar prophylactic phlebotomy schedules may be indicated in family members with fully saturated serum iron binding capacity.[7] Hemoglobin levels should be obtained before each phlebotomy and clinically acceptable levels should be maintained. Serum iron saturation should be measured periodically during both the corrective and maintenance phases of therapy. Normal values can usually be achieved in two to three years and then are maintained. Serum protein concentrations should be monitored. Depletion during the corrective phase is rarely a problem. In the other conditions cited, the intensity and/or duration of therapy may be more limited and should be individually determined.

Indications for Therapeutic Leukapheresis

Therapeutic removal of white blood cells (WBC) is potentially indicated when a rapid drop of a high peripheral WBC could prevent leukostatic phenomena. This problem occurs only in patients who have acute leukemia or aggressive myeloproliferative disorders. No set white blood cell count has been determined as a sign to initiate this procedure, but, as a rule of thumb, a count of over $100 \times 10^3/\text{cm}$ presents the danger of the patient having irreparable neurological damage secondary to the leukostatic phenomena can ensue. To obtain a sustained drop of the WBC, simultaneous treatment of the underlying disorder is of the essence. Adjuvant immunotherapy with allogeneic irradiated leukemic cells has been reported to have some success in increasing the survival of patients with acute myelogenous leukemia.[8]

Leukapheresis has been employed as the sole therapy to control the WBC in chronic myelogenous leukemia. No change in the natural course of the disease has been noted.[9] It may seem more rational to leukapherese patients with chronic lymphatic leukemia because the rate of cell proliferation is so low, and regression of adenopathy and organomegaly have

157

been reported, as well as, the lowering of WBC. There is, however, no evidence that the long natural course of the disease has been altered in any way and, therefore, leukapheresis must still be considered an investigational application.[10]

Indications for Therapeutic Plateletpheresis

Elevated platelet counts, usually twice normal values or more, may be associated with either abnormal bleeding or thrombotic phenomena. Reactive thrombocytosis seen with bleeding, inflammation or postsplenectomy is usually transient and rarely requires therapy. Thrombocytosis, as a feature of one of the myeloproliferative disorders, is often symptomatic and usually requires therapy.[11] Plateletpheresis repeated at 24- to 48-hour intervals can progressively lower the platelet count to clinically acceptable levels. The lowered platelet count response is transient and may be followed by a rebound rise so that plateletpheresis is usually employed as an adjunctive therapy or in emergency situations for short-term control of excessive thrombocytosis.

Indications for Therapeutic Exchange Plasmapheresis

Established

Paraproteinemias (Multiple Myeloma, Macroglobulinemia)

Plasma exchange is the treatment of choice when the symptomatology of these patients is presumed to be secondary to hyperviscosity. As a rule, patients are symptomatic when their serum viscosity is above 3 (relative to water at 37 C).[12] Plasma exchange is also indicated for patients who demonstrate hemostatic defects—eg, platelet dysfunction, or inhibition of coagulation factors—to stop the bleeding phenomena. Renal failure in these patients has been successfully treated with exchange plasmapheresis and diuresis in two instances; however, this application is still considered investigational. It should be kept in mind that this method of therapy is merely symptomatic and should be used at the time of diagnosis for immediate relief; at the same time specific therapy for the underlying disorder should commence.

Exchange plasmapheresis may be used as supportive therapy until chemotherapy has decreased the synthetic rate of the abnormal globulins. It should rarely serve as the sole modality of treatment in those cases when chemotherapy is either unsuccessful or cannot be tolerated by the patients. If more than one exchange is contemplated, the frequency of the procedures must be ascertained by doing serial determinations of the abnormal laboratory parameters following the initial procedure until baseline levels are reached. Symptomatic depletion of essential proteins has not been reported.

Cryoglobulinemia

Mixed cryoglobulins are thought to represent cold precipitable immune complexes. There is no known conventional therapy truly effective in this disease. Plasma exchange therapy is successful both in marked symptomatic relief and sizable decrease in circulating cryoglobulins.[13] Monthly exchanges of 2.5 liters have been successful in achieving a performance status of 100% in four cases treated in this fashion for five years or more.[14]

Thrombotic Thrombocytopenic Purpura (TTP)

Success in the treatment of this disorder has been uniformly reported when the replacement fluid is fresh frozen plasma (FFP).[15] There is some controversy as to whether FFP contains a factor in which these patients are deficient and whether this factor is responsible for the remission. Lian has presented data to support this in vivo, and one case has been reported involving relapse after plasma exchange and response to FFP infusion alone.[16] In one case, FFP was transfused to the point of volume overload and the patient failed to respond. Only repeated plasma exchanges ($\times$ 3) reversed the hematological changes. Today, the treatment of choice of thrombotic thrombocytopenic purpura is exchange plasmapheresis and antiplatelet drugs (eg, aspirin, and dipiridamol).

Goodpasture's Syndrome (Antibody-Mediated Nephritis and Lung Hemorrhage)

This disease has been successfully treated by Lockwood et al.[17] It was arrested particularly in those patients where pulmonary hemorrhage was an important clinical feature. Acutely deteriorating renal function was improved (fall in serum creatinine and disappearance of antiglomerular basement membrane antibody) even in patients that require dialysis. However, if the patients were anuric, no return of renal function occurred.

Investigational

Diseases of Excess Serum Components

Hyperlipidemias (Familial Hypercholesterolemia, Primary Biliary Cirrhosis, Diabetes)

Thompson et al[18] reported a loss of angina, reduced cholesterol, and low density lipoproteins when two 4.5-liter exchanges at three-week intervals were performed (two cases). In two additional cases, reported by Berger,[19] objective documentation of improvement (stress EKG) was obtained. Resolution of neuropathy and disappearance of xanthomata secondary to hyperlipemia in two cases of primary biliary cirrhosis was described by Turnberg et al.[20] The slow turnover of lipid pools probably contributes to the success of this modality of therapy.

Removal of Protein Bound Factors

Thyrotoxicosis

Thyrotoxicosis can usually be managed by conventional drug therapy but a few cases remain resistant to treatment. Several cases successfully treated with plasma exchange have been reported.[21] The potential benefit offered by plasma exchange lies in the fact that thyroid hormone is bound to plasma protein and, therefore, is potentially removable.

Poisons

Again, this treatment may be of value only when the ingested material is protein bound. Methyl parathion (a pesticide) and poisonous mushroom ingestion has been successfully treated in this fashion.[22,23]

Liver Failure

The presumption that some of the toxins responsible for coma are protein bound motivated several investigators to turn to exchange plasmapheresis.[24,25] The reported results were mixed.

Immunological Disorders

Neurological

Myasthenia Gravis

Understanding of the pathogenic mechanism of circulating antibody to the acetylcholine receptor has led to treating patients with therapeutic exchange plasmapheresis. Preliminary evidence[26] suggests the remission obtained by intensive plasmapheresis (5 to 10 consecutive procedures) can be maintained with subsequent judicious immunosuppressive therapy.

Amyotrophic Lateral Sclerosis

Norris et al[27] did a plasma exchange trial, acting on the possibility that immune complexes might play a role in this disease; however, no significant improvement was noted.

Guillain-Barré Syndrome

Because an IgM antibody is presumed to be important as a pathogenic agent, exchange plasmapheresis was tried in one case with a striking response.[28]

Hematological

Factor VIII Inhibitor

Antibodies to Factor VIII developing in hemophiliacs may present a major problem in management. Plasma exchange can satisfactorily extend the half-life of subsequently administered Factor VIII. This benefit is generally short term and can possibly be prolonged by immune suppressive therapy.[29]

Idiopathic Thrombocytopenic Purpura (ITP) and Autoimmune Hemolytic Anemia (AIHA)

Mixed reports on the effects of plasma exchange are available.[30,31] This is probably due to the fact that the pathogenic agents are IgG antibodies which have both an intra- and extravascular distribution and are more difficult to remove.

Hemolytic Disease of the Newborn (HDN)

Several workers have demonstrated that intensive exchange plasmapheresis started early (at the beginning of the second trimester of pregnancy) combined with intrauterine transfusions improves fetal survival in immunized mothers.[32]

Cold Agglutinin Disease

Theoretically, since the antibodies that cause the hemolytic anemia in this disease are of the IgM variety, this modality of therapy should be beneficial to the patients. However, in four cases, it was only successful when used as an adjuvant to chemotherapy (two cases). When used as a single modality of treatment, the benefit was of a very short duration (two cases).[33]

Dermatological

Pemphigus Vulgaris

These patients are reputed to have circulating antibody to intercellular epidermal cement substance. There are controversial reports regarding

161

efficacy of exchange plasmapheresis in the management of these patients. Furthermore, the lack of sensitivity of the antibody assay makes it impossible to correlate changes in titer with clinical response.[34]

Herpes Gestationis

One case was treated successfully when there was a clear-cut relationship in the decrease of the antibody against the basement membrane zone of normal skin (which is thought to have pathogenic significance) and the symptomatic improvement.[35]

Immune Complex Disorders (IC)

Currently, the largest growth in the application of exchange plasmapheresis is occurring in the field of immune complex disorders. The procedure is generally used in conjunction with cytotoxic and steroid drugs in an attempt to control immune complex formation.

Interpretation of the results of exchange plasmapheresis used in immune complex diseases is difficult because of the heterogenicity in the population of immune complexes and the lack of a clear relationship with the spectrum of disease activity. The different pharmacological agents these patients are receiving at the time exchange plasmapheresis is considered, make it practically impossible to evaluate the results. Some of these diseases are known to respond to conventional drugs and in some, spontaneous remissions are part of their natural history.

Systemic Lupus Erythematosus (SLE)

Verrier-Jones et al[36] have accumulated evidence that in patients with systemic lupus erythematosus who are deteriorating despite full doses of steroids and cytotoxic drugs, and who have high levels of circulating immune complexes, exchange plasmapheresis may produce a striking clinical and immunochemical improvement. Several other groups have experienced similar findings, namely, a linear relationship between the decrease of immune complexes and the favorable clinical course in progressive disease.

Wegener's Polyarteritis, Subacute Bacterial Endocarditis and Kidney Transplant Rejection

These three diseases have been treated with exchange plasmapheresis with reported success.[37-39]

Rheumatoid Arthritis

Several cases of rheumatoid arthritis have been treated effectively with exchange plasmapheresis by Wallace et al.[40] Reported remissions were sustained for an average of four months. All patients who experienced symptomatic relief were also taking gold or D-penicillamine concurrently.

Reports of single cases suffering from miscellaneous disorders successfully treated with plasma exchange include: bronchial asthma, hypertension, Guillain-Barré syndrome, and Raynaud's disease. Solid tumors have been treated with exchange plasmapheresis with varying degrees of success.[41]

Summary

The applications of exchange plasmapheresis are multiple. The diseases that have been managed in this fashion are varied and the number of diseases so managed is likely to increase. The efficacy of exchange plasmapheresis in producing symptomatic relief in paraproteinemia is indisputable, and the same can be stated for thrombotic thrombocytopenic purpura and Goodpasture's syndrome. The usefulness of exchange plasmapheresis in the other disorders mentioned is not completely documented and is still considered experimental. Exchange plasmapheresis is a benign procedure, with no side effects, when performed in a judicious manner. The questions of how much, when, and what is an ideal replacement fluid remain to be answered. Research on this modality of therapy is quite active, and, presumably, the answers will come in soon.

References

1. Dameshek, W: The case for phlebotomy in polycythemia vera: A panel discussion. *Blood* 32:488, 1968.
2. Wintrobe MM: *Clinical Hematology,* ed 7. Philadelphia, Lea & Febiger, 1974, chap 30.
3. Hurst JW, Spann JF: *Treatment of Heart Failure in the Heart,* ed 3. McGraw-Hill Book Co, 1974, p 487.
4. Williams R, Smith PM, Spicer EJF, et al: Venisection therapy in idiopathic hemochromatosis. *Q J Med* New series XXXVIII 149:1, 1969.
5. Epstein JH, Redeker AG: Porphyria cutanea tarda—a study of the effect of phlebotomy. *N Engl J Med* 279:1301, 1968.
6. Mollison PL: *Blood Transfusion in Clinical Medicine,* ed 5. Oxford, England, Blackwell Scientific Publications, 1972, p 616.
7. Cartwright GE: *Harrison's Principles of Internal Medicine,* ed 8. McGraw-Hill Book Company, 1977, p 652.
8. Oliver RTD, Lister TA, Russell J: Leucopheresis in the manage-

ment of patients with acute leukemia, in Goldman JM, Lowenthal RM (eds): *Leucocytes: Separation, Collection and Transfusion.* New York, Academic Press Inc., 1975, p 471.

9. Heustis DW, Price MJ, White RF, et al: Leukapheresis of patients with chronic granulocytic leukemia (CGL) using the Haemonetics Blood Processor. *Transfusion* 16:225, 1975.

10. Curtis JE, Hersh EM, Freireich EJ: Leukapheresis therapy of chronic lymphocytic leukemia. *Blood* 39:163, 1972.

11. Greenberg BR, Watson-Williams: Successful control of life-threatening thrombocytosis with a blood processor. *Transfusion* 15:620, 1975.

12. Russell JA, Toy JL, Powles RL: Plasma exchange in malignant paraproteinemia. *Exp Hematol* 5:105, 1977.

13. Lockwood CM: Plasma exchange in cryoglobulinemia. *Kidney Int,* to be published.

14. According to personal scientific experience by L. M. Reich, MD.

15. Bukowski, RM, King JW, Hewlett JS: Plasmapheresis in the treatment of thrombotic thrombocytopenic purpura. *Blood* 50:413, 1977.

16. Lian EC, Harkness DR, Byrnes JJ: Presence of a platelet aggregating factor in the plasma of patients with thrombotic thrombocytopenic purpura (TTP) and its inhibition by normal plasma. *Blood* 53:333, 1979.

17. Lockwood CM: The treatment of Goodpasture's syndrome and glomerulonephritis. *Plasma Therapy* 1:19, 1979.

18. Thompson GR, Lowenthal R, et al: Plasma exchange in the management of homozygous familial hypercholesterolemia. *Lancet* i:1208, 1975.

19. Berger GM, Miller JL, Bonniel F: Continuous flow plasma exchange in the treatment of homozygous familial hypercholesterolemia. *Am J Med* 65:243, 1978.

20. Turnberg LA, Mahoney MP, Gleeson MH: Plasmapheresis and plasma exchange in the treatment of hyperlipaemia and xanthomatous neuropathy in patients with primary biliary cirrhosis. *Gut* 13:976, 1972.

21. Horn K, Brehm G, Habermann J: Successful treatment of thyroid storm by continuous plasmapheresis with a blood cell separator. *Klin Wochenschr* 54:983, 1976.

22. Luzhnikov EA, Yaroslavsky AA, Molodenkov MN: Plasma perfusion through charcoal in methylparathion poisoning (letter). *Lancet* i:38, 1977.

23. Lembeck F: Elimination of toxic substances with marked plasma protein binding properties. *Wien Klin Wochenschar* 89:257, 1976.

24. Boland J, et al: Plasmapheresis in the treatment of fulminating hepatitis with coma. *Acta Clin Belg* 31:173, 1976.

25. Reich L, Turnbull A: Combined renal and hepatic failure. The potential of serial hemodialysis and massive exchange plasmapheresis. *Curr Prob Cancer* 4:18-20, 1979.

26. Lisak RP, Abramsky O, Schotland DL: Plasmapheresis in the treatment of myasthenia gravis. Preliminary studies in 21 patients, in *Plasmapheresis and the Immunobiology of Myasthenia Gravis.* Houghton Mifflin, 1978, p 209.

27. Norris RH, Denys EH, Mielke CH: Plasmapheresis in amyotrophic lateral sclerosis. *Muscle Nerv* I:342, 1978.

28. Brettle RP, Gross M, Legg N, et al: Treatment of acute polyneuropathy by plasma exchange. *Lancet* ii:1100, 1978.

29. Cobcroft R, Tamagnini G, Dormandy KM: Serial plasmapheresis in a haemophiliac with antibodies to Factor VIII. *J Clin Pathol* 30:763, 1977.

30. Branda RF, Moldas CF, McCullough JJ, et al: Plasma exchange in the treatment of immune disease. *Transfusion* 15:570, 1975.

31. Novak R, Williams J: Plasmapheresis in catastrophic complications of idiopathic thrombocytopenic purpura. *J Paed* 92:434, 1978.

32. Fraser ID, et al: Intensive antenatal plasmapheresis in severe rhesus isoimmunization. *Lancet* i:6, 1976.

33. Reich L: Personal experience.

34. Ruocco V, Rossi A, Argenziano G, et al: Pathogenicity of the intercellular antibodies of pemphigus and their periodic removal from the circulation by plasmapheresis. *Br J Dermatol* 98:237, 1978.

35. Lockwood CM: Plasma Exchange: An overview. *Plasma Therapy* 1:1, 1979.

36. Verrier-Jones J: Plasmapheresis in the management of systemic lupus erythematosis. *Muscle Nerv* 1:339, 1978.

37. Lockwood CM, et al: Plasma exchange in nephritis. *Adv Nephrol,* to be published.

38. Landwehr DM, Evans PS, et al: Removal of immune complexes by phasmapheresis in patients with subacute bacterial endocarditis. *Proc Int Cong Nephrol,* Abstr D33, 1978.

39. Cardella CJ, Sutton D, Uldall PR, et al: Intensive plasma exchange and renal transplant rejection. *Lancet* i:264, 1977.

40. Wallace DJ, Goldfinger D, et al: Plasmapheresis and lymphoplasmapheresis in the management of rheumatoid arthritis. *Arthritis Rheum* 22:703, 1979.

41. Hobbs JR, Byrom N, Elliot P, et al: Cell separators in cancer immunotherapy. *Exp Haematol* 5 Suppl:95, 1977.

Chapter 16

TRANSFUSION SERVICE LIABILITY

David E. Willett, JD

Introduction

THE HOSPITAL transfusion service—and its medical director—must be sensitive to legal requirements and potential liability. The most significant legal requirements are also requirements of good medical practice, since negligence is defined as a departure from those standards. Historically, negligence cases arising out of the transfusion service have most commonly involved errors in donor-recipient identification or pre-transfusion testing. However, transfusion service directors who accept greater responsibilities, such as participating more directly in diagnosis and treatment, greatly increase their potential liability. Omissions in the performance of administrative duties, such as the failure to take reasonable steps to assure an adequate supply of blood of an acceptable quality, may also be grounds for liability predicated on negligence. In addition to liability for negligence, transfusion service activities may provoke liability for the disregard of legally protected personal rights, or the violation of specific laws.

Negligence

Substandard conduct or error of omission is the most common basis for liability. Negligence is determined by measuring conduct against standards of good medical practice. A typical illustration can be found in *Parker v. Port Huron Hospital* (Mich. 1960), 105 N.W. 2d 1:

> "Certain pre-operative preparations were administered to Mrs. Parker the evening of her admission, including certain blood tests by Mrs. J.W., a laboratory technician in Port Huron Hospital Laboratory, to determine Mrs. Parker's blood type. Mrs. W. was the only laboratory technician working that evening. She testified that she was tired and overworked and that in drawing the blood sample from Mrs. Parker she didn't mark the patient's name or identification on the tube while at her bedside—she simply dropped a slip of paper around the tube. This procedure was contrary to universal standard practice required in this and other hospitals. On the same trip to Mrs. Parker's floor to obtain her blood sample, Mrs. W. had taken samples from two other patients. She returned to the laboratory with the three samples and commenced the work

167

of typing the samples, but was interrupted to do an immediate blood typing for a fourth patient. On her return to the work on the first three samples, she confused the sample tubes and the identification slips and designated Mrs. Parker's blood type as A-Rh positive rather than the correct blood type of O-Rh positive."

The patient received A-positive blood. Ultimately, she expired and the cause of death was reported as "acute nephrosis (lower hephron syndrome) incompatible blood transfusion." Incompatible blood transfusion is probably the most common cause for liability after transfusion, but a breach in any aspect of practice may be asserted as grounds for recovery.

In Chapter 1, the authors urge that the transfusion service medical director, in the interest of enhanced patient care, accept responsibility for all transfusions. Where the director actively participates in clinical decisions relating to transfusions, he necessarily assumes direct responsibility to the patient. That responsibility may also arise even though the director has not actively participated in the decision-making process, if the institution adopts formal routines and requirements for transfusion that make the director a constructive participant in each instance. If the transfusion service medical director accepts expanded responsibilities so that blood products are no longer "ordered," he must recognize that there is greater occasion for liability.

Even in institutions where the transfusion service medical director does not have the expanded responsibilities suggested in Chapter 1, the director is responsible to patients. When it appears that the patient's life or health may be threatened by a proposed transfusion, the medical director should take appropriate action. Liability might arise if the transfusion service medical director knew or should have known that an inappropriate transfusion was contemplated, and did nothing to intervene. Depending on the circumstances, the transfusion service medical director, at the least, may be held responsible for calling the attending physician's attention to potential consequences. Where transfusion is clearly inappropriate, the court is likely to conclude that the medical director has an obligation to withhold blood or otherwise see that the patient is protected. Common medical staff procedures should be used for this purpose.

In the administration of the transfusion, attention to the maintenance of a safe and adequate supply is important. Also, attention must be given to applicable standards of staffing, personnel qualifications, and training (including proficiency testing), record keeping, and equipment. For instance, in *Redding v. United States* (1961), 196 F. Supp. 871, a patient was given 1,000 cc of B-positive blood while in the operating room under anesthesia. Prior to surgery, the technician in this military hospital had typed and crossmatched the patient's blood as group B, Rh-positive. When complications arose, the Chief of the Laboratory Service was called. He testified:

> "I then went to the laboratory, where Pfc. L. and I rechecked the blood group and Rh type of the patient. On testing the specimen a number of times, we felt that the patient was either Group O, Rh-positive, or a very weak Group B, Rh-positive."

The patient was ultimately determined to be Group O, Rh-positive. The Government, defending the suit, contended that the pretransfusion error did not constitute negligence. The court dismissed this contention, and focused on the training of Sp-4 Doe, who had performed the crossmatch prior to transfusion.

> "In this connection it should also be borne in mind that Sp-4 Doe, prior to his entry in the Army on November 6, 1958, had only finished high school and attended a junior college for a period of one year. He was assigned to the hospital on January 3, 1959, for on-the-job training, and had been on the job training for eleven months when the mistake was made. . ."

The court contrasted his experience with the specialized education and training of his technician supervisor. Inadequate qualifications or training may tip the balance in close cases. Failure to participate in usual quality assurance activities also may invite questions as to the adequacy of supervision or management.

Strict Liability

There have been repeated efforts, since a New York case (Pearlmutter v. Beth David Hospital, 123 N.E. sd 792), to hold hospitals and physicans "strictly liable" for any injury attributable to blood transfusion. Most such cases have involved posttransfusion hepatitis. Whether called "strict liability in tort" or "implied warranty," the result would be the same. The transfusion service, hospital, or physician would be liable for the consequences, even in the absence of any negligence or fault. The threat of such liability has been minimized. Strict liability or implied warranty depends on the existence of a sale, and does not arise on the provision of a service. Most jurisdictions have adopted statutes, as the result of an American Association of Blood Banks' (AABB) campaign, which generally state that the provision of blood is not a sale of a commodity.

More recent examples of such legislation specifically provide that there shall be liability only for negligence in the provision of blood or its transfusion. Numerous recent attempts by attorneys representing plaintiffs to upset these statutes have been considered by both federal and state appellate courts. So far, these efforts have been unsuccessful. Liability without fault remains a concern in those few jurisdictions which have not adopted protective legislation, but case law weighs against such liability even in those states.

Constitutionally Protected Rights

Transfusion service medical directors may be involved in situations where a transfusion is medically necessary but is refused by the patient. Generally, such objections are on religious grounds, particularly if the patient is a Jehovah's Witness. Informed consent is usually a prerequisite for any medical procedure, and treatment ordinarily is not administered over a patient's objection. However, several court decisions indicate that patients may be required to accept blood transfusions in spite of religious objections. The courts will probably order transfusions for minors when parents refuse consent on religious grounds. (See *State v. Perricone* (1962) 181 A. 2d 751.)

Courts may also require pregnant patients to submit to transfusions if there is a threat to the life of the mother or the unborn child. (See *Raleigh Fitkin-Paul Morgan Memorial Hospital v. Anderson* (1964) 201 A. 2d 537). Even in the absence of pregnancy, adult patients may be required to accept blood over the objections of next-of-kin. In *John F. Kennedy Memorial Hospital v. Heston* (1971) 279 A. 2d 670, the court concluded that "there is no constitutional right to choose to die." The court reasoned:

> "Hospitals exist to aid the sick and injured. The medical and nursing professions are consecrated to preserving life. That is their professional creed. To them, a failure to use a simple, established procedure in the circumstances of this case would be malpractice, however the law may characterize that failure because of the patient's private convictions. A surgeon should not be asked to operate under the strain of knowing that a transfusion may not be administered even though medically required to save his patient. The hospital and its staff should not be required to decide whether the patient is or continues to be competent to make a judgment upon the subject, or whether the release tendered by the patient or a member of his family will protect them from civil responsibility. The hospital could hardly avoid the problem by compelling the removal of a dying patient, and Miss Heston's family made no effort to take her elsewhere.
>
> "When the hospital and staff are thus involuntary hosts and their interests are pitted against the belief of the patient, we think it reasonable to its staff to pursue their functions according to their professional standards. The solution sides with life, the conservation of which is, we think, a matter of state interest. A prior application

to a court is appropriate if time permits it, although in the nature of the emergency the only question that can be explored satisfactorily is whether death will probably ensue if medical procedures are not followed. If a court finds, as the trial court did, that death will likely follow unless a transfusion is administered, the hospital and the physician should be permitted to follow that medical procedure."

In such circumstances, a court order prior to transfusion is certainly desirable. The transfusion service medical director may prepare for such a contingency by requesting that hospital administration ask the hospital's attorney to determine how court approval can be obtained quickly. If there is no time to obtain a court order before administering blood, it is logical that the physicians and others participating should not be liable to the patient, even in jurisdictions where the courts have not resolved this issue.

Records

Good medical records are the key to successful liability defense. Keeping adequate records is a requirement of good medical practice, as well as a legal requirement. Failure to maintain necessary records may be actionable negligence in itself. Those records which should be maintained are described in the AABB *Standards for Blood Banks and Transfusion Services* and *Technical Manual,* and in federal and state laws and regulations. Routine hospital practices for making entries in medical records should be followed in the transfusion service. Corrections should be initialed, and original entries should not be obliterated when corrections are made. Records should be kept up to date, and entries should be made contemporaneously with the events recorded.

In *Pigno v. Bunim,* 350 NYS IId 438, liability was imposed upon a physician who could not substantiate his testimony with medical records. In that case, a complete blood exchange transfusion was necessary for an Rh-positive baby whose mother was Rh-negative. The process was halted after 120 cc of blood had been exchanged, because the baby became cyanotic. The exchange transfusion was not resumed until four days later. During that time, the baby developed deep jaundice and showed signs of kernicterus. The attending physician, Dr. S., testified that transfusion was postponed because the baby was still cyanotic. Imposing liability on Dr. S., the court reasoned:

"Dr. S. testified that bilirubin tests were of vital importance, that proper medical practice required the taking of such tests and that he had ordered the baby constantly monitored and bilirubin tests to be made every eight hours. The hospital records do not confirm that testimony. Furthermore, even assuming he had given such orders, a jury might find him remiss, as the physician in charge of the case, in failing to check that the orders were being carried out in an area as critical as this was.

"Physicians are not liable for mistakes in professional judgment, provided that they do what they think best after examination. However, liability can ensue if their judgment is not based upon intelligence and thus there is a failure to exercise any professional judgment.

"Giving plaintiff the benefit of all reasonable inferences, a jury could find that the decision to postpone the transfusion was not the result of careful analysis. There is no indication in the hospital records that plaintiff remained cyanotic; nor is there an indication that bilirubin tests were made every eight hours. The doctor's order sheet for plaintiff was missing from the hospital records. No results of such tests appeared in laboratory reports or in nurses' notes. Dr. S. apparently made no notation of the results of such tests or of their effect on the prescribed course of treatment."

In the absence of adequate records maintained in accordance with the standard of practice, unsubstantiated testimony may be doubted.

If a suit arises, no changes or additions should be made in existing records unless the reasons for the changes are first discussed with legal counsel. Otherwise, a jury may view the act as the admission of a guilty conscience, or as a record tampering.

Informed Consent, Releases, and Waivers

Record decisions in many jurisdictions deal with "informed consent" prior to medical treatment. Liability has been imposed for failure to secure informed consent. There is variation among states with respect to requirements of informed consent. Concern about potential liability has spawned a host of "consent forms," often embodying purported releases from any liability. In the opinion of this author, special consent forms for patients who may receive transfusions are unnecessary.

As a general proposition, the transfusion service medical director is responsible for securing informed consent only if he directly participates in the decision to transfuse. If that decision has been made by the attending physician, so that the transfusion service is asked only to furnish appropriate blood and to perform necessary laboratory work, the obligation to secure informed consent rests upon the attending physician.

Ordinarily, transfusion is incidental to some other procedure. The physician's obligation to secure informed consent to transfuse—and the extent of that obligation—depends on the circumstances of the case. Whether the physician has the obligation to advise the patient of the risk of hepatitis depends on the facts and on state law. Some courts may

172

conclude that this risk should be mentioned, particularly in elective procedures. Others have concluded differently, depending both on the factual circumstances and the law of the jurisdiction. Again, it must not be assumed that this duty rests on the transfusion service medical director.

Assuming that the law requires discussion of the risk of hepatitis, or other specific risks, a form is not necessarily a panacea. Too often, standardized forms are neither explained nor read. A form may be useful in documenting a discussion, but the physician's own testimony may be equally acceptable, particularly if documented by a simple chart note that indicates discussion of risks and alternatives. In a 1975 decision (*Sawyer v. Methodist Hospital of Memphis, Tennessee*), the United States Court of Appeals, discussing the informed consent issue, observed:

> "The likelihood of contracting hepatitis as a result of a blood transfusion is extremely remote. It appears that over the course of five or six years, about 60,000 units of blood were administered at Methodist Hospital with only eight cases of hepatitis apparently related to the transfusions—an incidence rate of .013%. In addition, hepatitis, although a serious illness, is not necessarily fatal and frequently responds to treatment. We believe that . . . this is not the kind or risk that defendants were bound to disclose before proceeding wth the transfusons."

Generally, it is overreaching on the part of the transfusion service to insist that specialized consent forms be executed prior to transfusion.

Occasionally, other special release forms have been utilized by transfusion services. Requests for uncrossmatched or partly processed blood in emergency situations have prompted the drafting of release forms, including assumptions of liability, to be signed by the requesting physician. Such forms consider the medical justification for proceeding in this manner, weighing potential adverse consequences against the asserted justification. Alternatives may be suggested. Generally, if the physician persists in his request, and if it is not clearly improper, blood should be furnished. At this point, the transfusion service medical director will want to document the circumstances supporting a departure from usual practice and standards, including necessary communications with the requesting physician.

Appropriate entries should be made in the records of the transfusion service. It is important that these entries be made contemporaneously with the event. The transfusion service may insist on a written request prior to releasing blood. However, the purpose of this request is to ensure that there is no misunderstanding, and to provide subsequent documentation. Insisting on the requesting physician's own signature on such a requisition may be impractical, particularly if he or she is scrubbed for surgery. Someone else in a position to verify the request may be asked to sign. The requesting physician may be asked to countersign the request as soon as possible.

Exculpatory language in such a form probably serves no useful purpose. It will not absolve the transfusion service medical director if, in fact, he has been derelict in considering the request. Such language may frighten the requesting physician sufficiently so that he reconsiders the request, but language of this nature put before a jury may also unfairly impair his case. If blood is furnished before usual testing procedures are accomplished, those procedures should be completed as soon as possible, and necessary followup insured. Complete documentation is imperative.

Liability to Donors

Donors, as well as patients, are entitled to due care, measured by standards of good medical practice. Obviously, blood cannot be drawn without consent. Consent should be documented by the donor's execution of an appropriate form. The donor's consent does not relieve those drawing his blood from the obligation to use due care, any purported "release" contained in the consent form probably has no legal effect.

In *Boll v. Sharp & Dohme, Inc.* (NY 1953), 121 NYS 2d 20, a paid donor who fainted and fell after being drawn was successful in setting aside a purported release. The court held that the transfusion service nonetheless had the duty to use reasonable care, including anticipating that the plaintiff might become faint, and therefore was required to take reasonable measures to protect him from injury in case he were to fall unconscious. Although donors are not "patients," they should be accorded the same rights, insofar as they are applicable. This includes the right to confidentiality of medical information. Such information should not be released except with consent, or pursuant to statute or regulation, or in response to subpoena. Internal "peer review" use, such as investigation of transfusion reactions, is permissible.

Therapeutic Pheresis

The performance of therapeutic pheresis procedures in the hospital transfusion service is less novel than a nonhospital transfusion service's decision to provide the same services. Nonetheless, the emergence of this type of therapy and the use of this modality for an increasing number of indications warrants specific comment. Obviously, both the indications for the procedure and the appropriateness of the procedure under specific circumstances are medical decisions.

174

It may be contended that the transfusion service medical director is a necessary participant in making these decisions. However, it is difficult to draw a line between the responsibility of the clinician ordering such therapy and the responsibility of the transfusion service medical director. It is extremely important that there be no gap attributable to misplaced reliance by one on the other. A protocol which recognizes and confirms the respective roles of those involved and which contains sufficient protection in terms of physician availability and other concerns is desirable.

As experimental procedures win acceptance, demand may arise for treatment which, when carefully considered, is recognized as inappropriate. Transfusion service medical directors, consistent with their own responsibilities, must exercise control over therapy which might have serious consequences. In addition to insuring that medical decisions are justified, it is desirable to assure that the medical record adequately supports those decisions. As in the case of any other medical procedure, informed consent is necessary. The manner in which obtaining consent is documented depends upon local law, the procedure and the circumstances. Here again those responsible for the procedure must insure that the patient receives the requisite explanation of risks and alternatives, and this aspect of the process must not fall between the cracks.

Legal concerns with respect to therapeutic pheresis center around adequate delineation of responsibilities, the recognition that the transfusion service medical director may be more directly involved than in other transfusion practices, and the establishment of backup procedures or other precautions, indicated whenever new procedures are offered. Obligations to pheresis donors are also important, particularly in the areas of informed consent, including informed consent to the administration of any medication.

Directors, and more than 50 committees of volunteer professionals.

AABB Purposes

...To function as a national association of hospital and community blood banks, transfusion and other immunohematologic services;

...To make available for the patient through blood banks a safe, adequate, economical and voluntary supply of whole blood or its components or derivations for the alleviation of pain and suffering and the saving of human lives;

...To encourage voluntary donation of blood and other tissues and organs through education, public information and research;

...To foster scientific investigation, clinical application, education and exchange of ideas and information relating to blood banks and transfusion services, as well as to other areas in the broad field of immunohematology, tissue and organ transplantation;

...To encourage, advance and certify high standards of administrative and technical performance in the general field of immunohematology as applied to blood banks, transfusion and/or transplantation services;

...To function as a national blood bank system or as a national blood bank system or available on a no-fee, 24-hour basis to assist in locating compatible blood for patients.

Any hospital or group of professional stature in the health professions, such as a national blood bank system or transfusion agency not located in the United States or its territories.

Individual Membership: Any individual whose qualifications satisfy one or more of the categories listed in the AABB Bylaws.

Sustaining Membership: Any member making an annual monetary contribution to the Association, equal to or exceeding the amount as determined by the Board, in addition to annual dues.

Services and Activities

Inspection and Accreditation Program, which, through the inspecting and accrediting of facilities, strives to improve the quality and safety of transfusions and assists the medical director of a blood bank or transfusion service in determining whether methods, procedures, and personnel meet established AABB standards. This voluntary service is offered without charge to member institutions. The I&A Program is recognized internationally as an educational tool to keep up-to-date on advances in research and technology. More than 550 blood bank professionals serve as volunteer inspectors. A number of

source of available rare blood types throughout the world. Listings are available on a no-fee, 24-hour basis to assist in locating compatible blood for patients.

Frozen Blood Depots ensure an immediate source of rare and super-rare blood.

Hepatitis B Surface Antigen Proficiency Testing Program is conducted with the College of American Pathologists on an annual subscription basis. It is designed to help laboratories attain and maintain a high quality of service.

Research in the many aspects of blood is carried out continuously by scientists and physicians associated with AABB at their local institutions. Their findings, shared at the AABB Annual Meeting and other prominent sessions and published in books and scientific journals, represent a major contribution to the advancement of medicine.

The AABB Research Foundation is a restricted endowment fund to encourage and foster the development of blood banking, scientific investigation, and clinical application in blood banking and blood transfusion therapy, immunohematology and organ and tissue transplantation. Donations and

aaBB

American Association of Blood Banks

The World's Leading Association for Blood Banking and Transfusion Therapy

About the AABB

Established in 1947, the American Association of Blood Banks is a professional, nonprofit scientific and administrative association for those individuals and institutions engaged in the many facets of blood banking. It is the only organization devoted exclusively to blood banking and blood transfusion services. AABB member facilities are responsible for collecting nearly half of the nation's blood supply and transfusing more than 80 percent. More than 2300 institutions (community and hospital blood banks and transfusion services) and 7000 individuals involved in blood banking are members of AABB, including physicians, scientists, medical technologists, administrators, blood donor recruiters and public-spirited citizens working with blood bankers. Members are located in all 50 states and 44 foreign countries. AABB's active membership gives direction to the Association through its Board of

Membership

There are four principal categories of membership:

Institutional Membership: Hospital and community blood banks and transfusion services engaged in the drawing of blood and other blood banking functions.

Associate Institutional Membership: Any hospital or group of professional stature in the health professions, committed to the concept of the voluntary donation of blood, which does not qualify for Institutional Membership.

...To function as a clearinghouse for the exchange of blood and blood credits on a local and nationwide basis;

...To plan for cooperation between blood banks and transfusion services in times of disaster.

National Clearinghouse Program provides a mechanism for the transfer of blood and blood credits between facilities across the country, thus allowing for the best possible utilization of blood resources. The Clearinghouse enables a blood donor to give blood in one part of the country for a patient receiving blood in another area.

Standby Contract with the Department of Defense systemizes procurement of blood by AABB banks in times of national emergency.

Reference Laboratories provide exchange of information and consultation on rare blood group antibodies, typing, crossmatching, component preparation and therapy, blood compatibility testing and research.

states accept AABB inspections as equivalent to their state licensing requirements.